Nutrition Services in Perinatal Care

SECOND EDITION

Committee on Nutritional Status During
Pregnancy and Lactation
Food and Nutrition Board
Institute of Medicine
National Academy of Sciences

National Academy Press
Washington, D.C. 1992

NATIONAL ACADEMY PRESS • 2101 Constitution Avenue, N.W. • Washington, DC 20418

NOTICE: The project that is the subject of this report was approved by the Governing Board of the National Research Council, whose members are drawn from the councils of the National Academy of Sciences, the National Academy of Engineering, and the Institute of Medicine. The members of the committee responsible for the report were chosen for their special competences and with regard for appropriate balance.

This report has been reviewed by a group other than the authors according to procedures approved by a Report Review Committee consisting of members of the National Academy of Sciences, the National Academy of Engineering, and the Institute of Medicine.

The Institute of Medicine was chartered in 1970 by the National Academy of Sciences to enlist distinguished members of the appropriate professions in the examination of policy matters pertaining to the health of the public. In this, the Institute acts under both the Academy's 1863 congressional charter responsibility to be an adviser to the federal government and its own initiative in identifying issues of medical care, research, and education.

This study was supported by project no. MCJ 117018 from the Maternal and Child Health Program (Title V, Social Security Act), Health Resources and Services Administration, U.S. Department of Health and Human Services.

Library of Congress Catalog Card No. 92-60920

International Standard Book Number 0-309-04694-7

Additional copies of this report are available for sale from:

National Academy Press
2101 Constitution Avenue, NW
Washington, DC 20418

S553

Printed in the United States of America

The serpent has been a symbol of long life, healing, and knowledge among almost all cultures and religions since the beginning of recorded history. The image adopted as a logotype by the Institute of Medicine is based on a relief carving from ancient Greece, now held by the Staatlichemuseen in Berlin.

First Printing, July 1992
Second Printing, January 1993

COMMITTEE ON NUTRITIONAL STATUS DURING PREGNANCY AND LACTATION

ROY M. PITKIN (*Chair*),* Department of Obstetrics and Gynecology, School of Medicine, University of California, Los Angeles, California
BARBARA ABRAMS, Program in Public Health Nutrition, School of Public Health, University of California, Berkeley, California
LINDSAY H. ALLEN, Department of Nutritional Sciences, University of Connecticut, Storrs, Connecticut
MARGIT HAMOSH, Division of Developmental Biology and Nutrition, Georgetown University Medical Center, Washington, D.C.
JANET C. KING, Department of Nutritional Sciences, University of California, Berkeley, California
CHARLES MAHAN, Department of Health and Rehabilitative Services, State Health Office, Tallahassee, Florida
JAMES MARTIN, Department of Obstetrics and Gynecology, University of Mississippi Medical Center, Jackson, Mississippi
CHRISTINE OLSON, Division of Nutritional Sciences, Cornell University, Ithaca, New York
LINDA A. RANDOLPH, Department of Community Medicine, Mount Sinai School of Medicine, on assignment to Carnegie Corporation of New York, New York, New York
KATHLEEN M. RASMUSSEN, Division of Nutritional Sciences, Cornell University, Ithaca, New York
JOHN W. SPARKS, Department of Pediatrics, University of Texas, Houston, Texas

Staff

CAROL WEST SUITOR, Study Director
YVONNE L. BRONNER, Research Associate (until July 1991)
SHEILA MYLET, Research Associate
GERALDINE KENNEDO, Administrative Assistant

*Member, Institute of Medicine

Staff

CATHERINE E. WOTEKI, Director
MARCIA LEWIS, Administrative Assistant
SUSAN WYATT, Financial Associate

Acknowledgments

The committee wishes to express its appreciation to the many people who made important contributions to this report by providing source materials or special written reports, sharing their views during workshops, commenting on drafts, or otherwise serving as resource persons. In particular, the committee wishes to thank David H. Adamkin, Department of Pediatrics, University of Louisville, Louisville, Ky.; Diane M. Anderson, Medical University of South Carolina, Charleston, S.C.; Cheryl Bowen, Maryland Institute for Emergency Medical Services Systems, University of Maryland, Baltimore, Md.; Mary Sue Brady, Department of Nutrition and Dietetics, Indiana University School of Medicine, Indianapolis, Ind.; Helen Varney Burst, Nurse Midwifery Program, Yale University, New Haven, Conn.; Jennifer Burton, Nurses Association of the American College of Obstetricians and Gynecologists, Washington, D.C.; Ronald Chez, Department of Obstetrics and Gynecology, University of South Florida, Tampa, Fla.; Julie A. Clapp, Delaware Health and Social Services, Dover, Del.; Harriet H. Cloud, Nutrition Division, Sparks Center for Developmental and Learning Disorders, University of Alabama, Birmingham, Ala.; Garris Keels Conner, National Association of Neonatal Nurses, Birmingham, Ala.; Susan Conner, County of Riverside Department of Health, Riverside, Calif.; Carlyle Crenshaw, Jr., Department of Obstetrics and Gynecology, University of Maryland Hospital, Baltimore, Md.; Katherine Davis, University of Mississippi Medical Center, Jackson, Miss.; Diane Dimperio, Department of Obstetrics and Gynecology, University of Florida, Gainesville, Fla.; Judith A. Ernst, Department of

Nutrition and Dietetics, Indiana University School of Medicine, Indianapolis, Ind.; S. Ann Evans, American Association of Critical-Care Nurses, Aliso Viejo, Calif.; Walter Faubion, University of Michigan Medical Center, Ann Arbor, Mich.; Ann M. Ferris, Department of Nutritional Sciences, University of Connecticut, Storrs, Conn.; Kyle Grazier, School of Public Health, University of California, Berkeley, Calif.; Robert Graham, American Academy of Family Physicians, Kansas City, Mo.; Erica Gunderson, Children's Hospital of San Francisco, San Francisco, Calif.; Ronald Gutberlet, Department of Pediatrics, Mercy Medical Center, University of Maryland, Baltimore, Md.; Gordon L. Klein, University of Texas Medical Branch, Child Health Center, Galveston, Tex.; Ronald E. Kleinman, Massachusetts General Hospital, Boston, Mass.; Becky Klingbail, University of Louisville, Louisville, Ky.; Winston Koo, University of Tennessee, Memphis, Tenn.; Ann Koontz, Maternal and Child Health Bureau, Hyattsville, Md.; Michele Lawler, Food and Nutrition Service, U.S. Department of Agriculture (USDA); James A. Lemons, Riley Newborn Follow-up Program, Indiana University School of Medicine, Indianapolis, Ind.; Brenda Lisi, Food and Nutrition Service, USDA, Alexandria, Va.; Gerald B. Merenstein, University of Colorado, Denver, Colo.; Renee McCleery, University of Texas Medical Branch, Galveston, Tex.; Laurie J. Moyer-Mileur, Nutrition Research, University of Utah, Salt Lake City, Utah; Sue Murvich, Lutheran Hospital, La Crosse, Wis.; Betty Jo Nelsen, Food and Nutrition Service, USDA, Alexandria, Va.; Stephanie Phelps, University of Tennessee, Memphis, Tenn.; Karyl Rickard, Department of Nutrition and Dietetics, Indiana University, Indianapolis, Ind.; Sandra Robbins, George Washington University Medical Center, Washington, D.C.; Helen Schauffler, School of Public Health, University of California, Berkeley, Calif.; Shirley Shelton, American College of Obstetricians and Gynecologists, Washington, D.C.; Melody Thompson, Children's Hospital, Columbus, Ohio; Jacqueline Jones Wessel, Children's Hospital Medical Center, Cincinnati, Ohio; Catherine W. Wiggins, National Association of Neonatal Nurses, Washington, D.C.; and Debra Wilson, University of Michigan Medical Center, Ann Arbor, Mich.

In particular, the committee wishes to acknowledge the essential role of the project director, Carol Suitor, in the development of this report. Without her assistance throughout the span from conception to printing, it could not have been done. Thanks also to many other staff members of the Food and Nutrition Board, the Institute of Medicine, and the Academy Complex, especially Catherine E. Woteki, Geraldine Kennedo, Yvonne Bronner, Sheila Mylet, Susan Wyatt, Sally Stanfield, and Leah Mazade.

Contents

List of Tables and Charts

Tables

Charts

Executive Summary

In 1988, the Food and Nutrition Board's Committee on Nutritional Status During Pregnancy and Lactation was constituted to reexamine important questions relating to nutritional care of pregnant and lactating women and their infants. The committee's work has been supported by the Maternal and Child Health Program (Title V, Social Security Act) of the U.S. Department of Health and Human Services. Together with three of its subcommittees, this broadly based committee issued *Nutrition During Pregnancy* and *Nutrition During Lactation*, thoroughly researched reports that present the committee's findings and recommendations in these areas. Subsequently, the committee's joint effort with a fourth subcommittee resulted in the publication *Nutrition During Pregnancy and Lactation: An Implementation Guide*, which is intended to help health care providers apply the recommendations made in the first two reports.

Because it was recognized that the actual application of recommendations and guidelines in specific care settings would require administrative support and possibly some organizational changes, the committee was also charged with revising the 1981 publication *Nutrition Services in Perinatal Care*. That first edition covered prenatal, postpartum, and neonatal nutrition services—including the personnel, competency levels, and support necessary to provide the services in a regionalized perinatal care system. This second edition updates the coverage of nutrition and nutrition services in a manner that would be applicable regardless of the system of care. Moreover, it expands the coverage of nutrition services for two important periods that received little attention previously: preconception and lactation. This edition also focuses increased attention on the rationale for the recommended nutrition services.

PREVIOUS RECOMMENDATIONS AND UNDERLYING ASSUMPTIONS

Relevant content and recommendations from *Nutrition During Pregnancy*, *Nutrition During Lactation*, and *Recommended Dietary Allowances* (another recent Food and Nutrition Board publication) are incorporated in this book. In addition, the committee agreed that the following assumptions would guide its work:

- A patient-centered, individualized approach promotes high-quality nutritional care.
- The development of nutritional care plans is a key element of nutrition services.
- Supportive family members or friends should be involved in the development and implementation of the nutritional care plan.
- A team effort enhances nutritional care, especially if health, economic, or social problems are involved.
- Efforts should be made to promote continuity of nutritional care.

OVERVIEW

The second edition of *Nutrition Services in Perinatal Care* describes two basic types of nutrition services: (1) *basic nutrition services*, which should be available to all women and infants in the course of usual health care, and (2) *special nutrition services*, which should be provided to women with health problems that complicate their nutritional care, to preterm infants, and to full-term infants with serious health problems. *Basic nutrition services* that address the mother's nutritional needs include early identification of women at risk for nutrition-related health problems, health maintenance activities for promoting adequate nutrition, and, as needed, basic nutrition interventions including counseling, food or vitamin-mineral supplementation, support, and referrals. *Special nutrition services*, which address complex nutritional problems related to medical or surgical conditions, usually require that a nutrition specialist, ordinarily an experienced registered dietitian, serve on the health care team. Examples of such health problems include insulin dependent diabetes mellitus, severe gastrointestinal disorders, and phenylketonuria; other examples are provided in the text.

CONTENTS OF THE REPORT

The seven chapters are organized as follows:

1. introductory material;
2. a brief review of the nutritional concerns of women in the preconceptional, prenatal, and postpartum periods—including the reasons selected health problems call for special nutrition services;
3. elements of basic and special nutrition services for women during the three periods mentioned above;
4. nutrition services for newborn infants, with a new focus on supporting breastfeeding;
5. elements of special nutrition services for preterm and sick newborns, prefaced by brief descriptions of the challenges such infants present and the feeding methods available; the chapter also includes a summary of the importance and complexity of monitoring;
6. an entirely new chapter on strategies for promoting the continuity of nutritional care; and
7. further comments and the committee's recommendations, the highlights of which are given below.

RECOMMENDATIONS

This report presents eight key recommendations:

- Basic, patient-centered, individualized nutritional care should be integrated into the primary care of every woman and infant—beginning prior to conception and extending throughout the period of breastfeeding.
- All primary care providers should have the knowledge and skills necessary to screen for nutritional problems, assess nutritional status, provide basic nutritional guidance, and implement basic nutritional care.
- Nutritional care should be documented in the permanent medical record.
- When health problems that benefit from special nutritional care are identified, there should be consultation with and often referral to an experienced registered dietitian or other appropriate specialists.
- Attention should be directed toward aspects of nutritional care that have been seriously neglected in the past: providing care prior to conception and in support of breastfeeding, and ensuring the continuity of nutritional care despite changes in providers.

- Action should be taken to make appropriate policy and structural changes for the promotion and support of breastfeeding.
- Where not already in place, mechanisms should be established to pay for basic and special nutrition services in both the public and the private sectors.
- Cost-effective strategies for implementing the nutritional care recommended in this report should be developed and tested.

1

Introduction

Nutrition plays a major role in promoting maternal and infant health.[1-6] Both the U.S. Preventive Services Task Force[7] and the Expert Panel on the Content of Prenatal Care[8] identify nutrition services as an essential component of prenatal care. This view is supported and expanded by the attention given to the nutrition of mothers and newborn infants in *Guidelines for Perinatal Care*,[9] a joint publication of the American Academy of Pediatrics and the American College of Obstetricians and Gynecologists.

The goal of this document is to help those responsible for the health care of women and infants to understand the rationale for nutrition services and to incorporate appropriate nutrition services into their care delivery system.

A growing body of evidence indicates tangible health benefits and possibly economic benefits of nutrition services during pregnancy[10,11] and the first year after birth. A few examples follow:

- The prenatal benefits of the Supplemental Food Program for Women, Infants, and Children (WIC)[a] may reduce the percentage of

---

[a]For an annotated bibliography on studies about the Supplemental Food Program for Women, Infants, and Children, see the Food Research and Action Center report *WIC: A Success Story*.[12] WIC offers three kinds of important benefits to eligible low-income individuals: access to a monthly package of highly nutritious supplemental foods, nutrition education and counseling to help participants become more aware of the role nutrition plays in achieving health and well-being, and referrals.

infants born with low birth weight; this, in turn, may produce substantial savings in Medicaid costs for newborns and their mothers.[13-15]

- Comprehensive nutritional care contributes to the survival of low birth weight and sick infants[16] (see Chapter 5).
- Postpartum participation in WIC may reduce the risk of low birth weight in subsequent pregnancies.[17]
- Home health visits with a nutrition component may contribute to earlier discharge of very-low-birth-weight infants.[18]

In some situations, the reduction in the number of low-birth-weight infants requiring expensive care in the hospital may offset the costs of prenatal nutrition counseling.[19]

Other studies[20-23] suggest that comprehensive care[b] improves pregnancy outcomes such as birth weight, especially for high-risk women[23] and for primiparous women,[22] and that it reduces complications for women with preexisting diabetes mellitus and their infants.[24] It is not clear, however, to what extent the nutrition services that were part of such care contributed to the improved outcomes.

BACKGROUND INFORMATION

The Food and Nutrition Board's Committee on Nutritional Status During Pregnancy and Lactation considered it important to revise the board's 1981 report *Nutrition Services in Perinatal Care*[25] to be consistent with current recommendations for nutritional care. It also sought to provide expanded coverage of the preconceptional period and of breastfeeding, and to make the report adaptable to different systems of care delivery. For this revision, three documents from the National Academy of Sciences and the Institute of Medicine (IOM) provide much of the scientific foundation for its content: the 1989 revision of *Recommended Dietary Allowances*,[26] *Nutrition During Pregnancy*,[5] and *Nutrition During Lactation*.[6]

The expanded coverage of preconceptional nutrition in this second edition of *Nutrition Services in Perinatal Care* is consistent with one of the main messages in *Caring for Our Future: The Content of Prenatal Care*[8] and with the increased attention to this period now being given by the American College of Obstetricians and Gynecologists and other professional organizations. Similarly, the increased emphasis on breastfeeding is

---

[b]Comprehensive care constitutes an array of supportive services, one of which is nutrition services.

a logical consequence of activities (including many research projects) that were stimulated by the Surgeon General's Workshop on Breastfeeding and Human Lactation.[27,28] This revision retains the original title even though the book now covers a period that extends well beyond that encompassed by the traditional definition of *perinatal*.

The first edition of *Nutrition Services in Perinatal Care* was written to identify "the personnel, competency levels, and support necessary to provide nutritional assessment and education and services within . . . a regionalized system" of perinatal care (p. 1).[25] In recognition of the current debate about the benefits[29-34] and evolution[34-38] of regionalized systems of perinatal care, this revised report was designed to be relevant, regardless of the system of perinatal care that is in place. New information about these systems may be forthcoming from the National Perinatal Information Center and the National Foundation, March of Dimes, both of which have been examining how regionalized systems have fared and what changes are indicated. In the meantime, *Guidelines for Perinatal Care*[9] addresses the current regionalized perinatal care system in detail.

During this period of transition in the delivery of regionalized perinatal care, changes have been occurring in the content of nutritional care for pregnant and lactating women and their infants, the sites at which such care is delivered, the personnel involved, and the ethnic composition of the populations that are served. Some of these changes have resulted from the growth of the Special Supplemental Food Program for Women, Infants, and Children,[c] the increase in the number of dietitians[d] available to provide nutrition counseling services upon referral, numerous technological developments in caring for very premature infants, increased immigration of Hispanics and Southeast Asians to the United States, and, most recently, the development of mechanisms for the reimbursement of nutrition services through Medicaid.[39-41] Moreover, the challenge of providing adequate nutrition services for pregnant migrant workers and homeless women is of growing concern.[42,43]

---

[c]In 1990, WIC served approximately 2,447,000 women and infants under the age of 1 year–2.4 times as many as it did in 1981 (J. Hirschman, Food and Nutrition Service, USDA, personal communication, 1991).

[d]In this document, the term *dietitian* is used to represent a qualified nutrition professional, ordinarily a registered or licensed dietitian or a nutritionist who is eligible for registration.

STUDY APPROACH AND SCOPE

The committee conducted an extensive search of the literature concerning regionalized perinatal care and nutrition services during the preconceptional, prenatal, postpartum, and neonatal periods. It requested and received written comments on the first edition of *Nutrition Services in Perinatal Care*[25] from a variety of organizations and content experts, and it supplemented these responses with a workshop to examine directions that the revision might take and to seek additional input from organizations. After deliberating and making revisions, the committee sought additional assistance and comments from health care providers and government agencies.

Two of the publications on which this book is based—*Nutrition During Pregnancy*[5] and *Nutrition During Lactation*[6]—make it clear that optimal nutritional care of women before, during, and after pregnancy is assessment based. That is, recommendations on nutrition are based on the interpretation of findings from the woman's history and physical examination. Thus, this revision of *Nutrition Services in Perinatal Care* develops the theme that there are two levels of nutritional care—basic and special—and that the level of care required by an individual is determined by the assessment. Chart 1-1 gives characteristics of these two levels of care.

The theme of two levels of nutritional care was also used in developing a companion document to the two IOM reports noted above. That document, *Nutrition During Pregnancy and Lactation: An Implementation Guide*,[44] presents information in a practical form to assist those involved in the delivery of basic nutritional care to expectant and new mothers. The document was developed by the Subcommittee for a Clinical Applications Guide in collaboration with this committee; its purpose is to translate the recommendations from the recent IOM reports *Nutrition During Pregnancy*[5] and *Nutrition During Lactation*[6] into a form that can be applied easily in the clinical setting. Consequently, such content is excluded from this revised edition.

The second edition of *Nutrition Services in Perinatal Care* focuses on nutrition services beginning in the preconceptional period and extending well beyond birth, and it gives the rationale for recommending that such services be provided. It briefly describes the necessary elements of these services and indicates the personnel and the knowledge, skills, and specialized education or training that may be needed to deliver them. It is not intended to set standards of care. However, it should prove useful to policymakers, hospital administrators, directors of health centers, physicians in private or group practice, and others responsible for setting such standards and for overseeing health care services for expectant and new mothers and their infants.

CHART 1-1 Characteristics of Basic and Special Nutrition Services

	Type of Nutritional Care	
	Basic	Special
Provider	Primary care providers such as physicians, midwives, nurse practitioners	A multidisciplinary team that includes an experienced dietitian or other nutrition-related specialists
Recipients	All women receiving preconceptional care All expectant mothers All infants	Women or infants with health conditions that affect dietary intake, digestion, or the absorption, utilization, or excretion of nutrients
Elements of care	Early identification of nutritional risk factors Core provision of health maintenance activities, such as education about pregnancy weight gain or breastfeeding Implementation of common interventions Follow-up of basic care	Basic care plus intensive nutrition services (e.g., detailed assessments, complex diet modifications, diet counseling, close monitoring, extended follow-up)

PREVIOUSLY PUBLISHED RECOMMENDATIONS AND UNDERLYING ASSUMPTIONS

In addition to accepting the recommendations of the previous IOM reports, the committee agreed that the following principles and philosophies would guide its work.

Patient-Centered, Individualized Care

A patient-centered, individualized approach promotes high-quality nutritional care. This means that a nutritional assessment should precede decisions concerning nutritional care. As used in this book, the term *nutritional assessment* covers a wide range of activities, not all of which are appropriate for all individuals. The measurement of height or length and weight, the determination of hemoglobin values, and the assessment of dietary practices are components of basic nutritional assessment for all. Abnormal findings may indicate the need for more thorough assessment and sometimes for intensive nutritional care.

Family Involvement in Care

Ideally, nutritional care for pregnant women and their infants involves supportive networks of people; often these people are family members and friends. Support from significant others may have a strong impact on how well the woman, her infant, or both are nourished.

Team Care

A team effort enhances nutritional care, just as it does other aspects of health care. The committee takes the position that the physician or midwife[e] is responsible for ensuring that nutrition services are provided as an integral aspect of health care and that various team members, with proper training, can provide basic nutrition services. The dietitian may serve either as a team member or as a resource person (i.e., to provide training and consultation to the health care providers, as well as direct nutritional services to women requiring special nutritional care). The specific roles of the dietitian will depend on how care is organized within the setting and on the complexity of the nutrition problem.

Continuity of Care

Continuity of nutritional care comprises many elements: consistency in the guidance provided by different team members, avoidance of dup-

---

[e]In this document, the term *midwife* is used to represent a qualified licensed midwife, ordinarily a certified nurse-midwife.

licated activities, a clear progression of care as the woman moves from the preconceptional period through pregnancy and breastfeeding, and building on previous nutritional care if the woman changes providers for any reason. It is assumed that efforts to promote continuity of nutritional care will enhance its quality.

ORGANIZATION OF THE REPORT

Throughout this book, distinctions are made between basic and special nutrition services. Chapter 2 provides the rationale for both kinds of nutrition services in the preconceptional, prenatal, and postpartum periods; it also provides a brief review of changes in maternal nutrient needs during those periods. The preconceptional and postpartum periods receive more detailed coverage than in the first edition. Chapter 3 describes the basic and special services that should be available to women in the preconceptional, prenatal, and postpartum periods; the respective personnel requirements; and the knowledge base and clinical skills required for both levels of care. Chapter 4 addresses the basic nutrition services needed for healthy neonates, for older infants who have been discharged from special care, and for mothers or other caregivers responsible for feeding such infants. Chapter 5 deals with the special nutrition services required by high-risk neonates and those responsible for their care. Chapter 6 summarizes three approaches that hold promise for improved continuity of nutritional care for mothers and their infants. Finally, Chapter 7 presents further comments and the committee's recommendations.

REFERENCES

1. Institute of Medicine. 1985. Preventing Low Birthweight. Report of the Committee to Study the Prevention of Low Birthweight, Division of Health Promotion and Disease Prevention. National Academy Press, Washington, D.C.
2. Department of Health and Human Services. 1988. The Surgeon General's Report on Nutrition and Health. DHHS (PHS) Publ. No. 88-50210. Public Health Service. U.S. Government Printing Office, Washington, D.C.
3. Department of Health and Human Services. 1990. Healthy People 2000: National Health Promotion and Disease Prevention Objectives. DHHS (PHS) Publ. No. 91-50212. Public Health Service, Office of the Assistant Secretary for Health, Washington, D.C.
4. Farthing, M.A.C., and M. Kaufman. 1990. Serving women, infants, and children. Pp. 139-171 in M. Kaufman, ed. Nutrition in Public Health. Aspen Publishers, Inc., Rockville, Md.
5. Institute of Medicine. 1990. Nutrition During Pregnancy: Weight Gain and Nutrient Supplements. Report of the Subcommittee on Nutritional Status and Weight Gain During Pregnancy and the Subcommittee on Dietary Intake and Nutrient Supplements During

Pregnancy, Committee on Nutritional Status During Pregnancy and Lactation, Food and Nutrition Board. National Academy Press, Washington, D.C.

6. Institute of Medicine. 1991. Nutrition During Lactation. Report of the Subcommittee on Nutrition During Lactation, Committee on Nutritional Status During Pregnancy and Lactation, Food and Nutrition Board. National Academy Press, Washington, D.C.
7. U.S. Preventive Services Task Force. 1989. Guide to Clinical Preventive Services. Williams & Wilkins, Baltimore, Md.
8. Department of Health and Human Services. 1989. Caring for Our Future: The Content of Prenatal Care. A Report of the Public Health Service Expert Panel on the Content of Prenatal Care. Public Health Service, Washington, D.C.
9. American Academy of Pediatrics/American College of Obstetricians and Gynecologists. 1992. Guidelines for Perinatal Care, 3rd ed. American Academy of Pediatrics, Elk Grove, Ill.
10. Disbrow, D.D. 1989. The costs and benefits of nutrition services: a literature review. II. Ambulatory nutrition care: pregnant women. J. Am. Diet. Assoc. 89 (4, suppl.):S10-S14.
11. Trouba, P.H., N. Okereke, and P.L. Splett. 1991. Summary document of nutrition intervention in prenatal care. J. Am. Diet. Assoc. 91 (11, suppl.):S21-26.
12. Food Research and Action Center. 1991. WIC: A Success Story, 3rd ed. Food Research and Action Center, Washington, D.C.
13. Devaney, B., L. Bilheimer, and J. Schore. 1990. The Savings in Medicaid Costs for Newborns and Their Mothers from Prenatal Participation in the WIC Program. 281-075/20915. Food and Nutrition Service, Office of Analysis and Evaluation, U.S. Department of Agriculture. U.S. Government Printing Office, Washington, D.C.
14. New York State Department of Health. 1990. The New York State WIC Evaluation: The Association Between Prenatal WIC Participation and Birth Outcomes. New York State Department of Health, Albany, N.Y.
15. Stockbauer, J. 1987. WIC prenatal participation and its relation to pregnancy outcomes in Missouri: a second look. Am. J. Public Health 77:813-818.
16. Heird, W.C., and A. Cooper. 1988. Nutrition in infants and children. Pp. 944-968 in M.E. Shils and V.R. Young, eds. Modern Nutrition in Health and Disease. 7th ed. Lea and Febiger, Philadelphia.
17. Caan, B., D.M. Horgen, S. Margen, J.C. King, and N.P. Jewell. 1987. Benefits associated with WIC supplemental feeding during the interpregnancy interval. Am. J. Clin. Nutr. 45:29-41.
18. Brooten, D., S. Kumar, L.P. Brown, P. Butts, S.A. Finkler, S. Bakewell-Sachs, A. Gibbons, and M. Delivoria-Papadopoulos. 1986. A randomized clinical trial of early hospital discharge and home follow-up of very-low-birth-weight infants. N. Engl. J. Med. 315:934-939.
19. Orstead, C., D. Arrington, S.K. Kamath, R. Olson, and M.B. Kohrs. 1985. Efficacy of perinatal nutrition counseling: weight gain, infant birth weight, and cost-effectiveness. J. Am. Diet. Assoc. 85:40-45.
20. Buescher, P.A., and N.I. Ward. 1992. A comparison of low birth weight among Medicaid patients of public health departments and other providers of prenatal care in North Carolina and Kentucky. Public Health Rep. 107:54-59.
21. Korenbrot, C.C. 1984. Risk reduction in pregnancies of low-income women. Mobius 4:34-43.
22. McLaughlin, F.J., W.A. Altemeier, M.J. Christensen, K.B. Sherrod, M.S. Dietrich, and D.T. Stern. 1992. Randomized trial of comprehensive prenatal care for low-income women: effect on infant birth weight. Pediatrics 89:128-132.
23. Taren, D.L., and S.N. Graven. 1991. The association of prenatal nutrition and educational services with low birth weight rates in a Florida program. Public Health Rep. 106:426-436.

24. Scheffler, R.M., L.B. Feuchtbaum, and C.S. Phibbs. 1992. Prevention: the cost-effectiveness of the California Diabetes and Pregnancy Program. Am. J. Public Health 82:168-175.
25. National Research Council. 1981. Nutrition Services in Perinatal Care. Committee on Nutrition of the Mother and Preschool Child, Food and Nutrition Board, Assembly of Life Sciences. National Academy Press, Washington, D.C.
26. National Research Council. 1989. Recommended Dietary Allowances, 10th ed. Report of the Subcommittee on the Tenth Edition of the RDAs, Food and Nutrition Board, Commission on Life Sciences. National Academy Press, Washington, D.C.
27. Department of Health and Human Services. 1984. Report of the Surgeon General's Workshop on Breastfeeding and Human Lactation. DHHS Publ. No. HRS-D-MC 84-2. Health Resources and Services Administration, Public Health Service, Rockville, Md.
28. Spisak, S., and S.S. Gross. 1991. Second Followup Report: The Surgeon General's Workshop on Breastfeeding and Human Lactation. National Center for Education in Maternal and Child Health, Washington, D.C.
29. Burkett, M.E. 1989. The tertiary center and health departments in cooperation: the Duke University experience. J. Perinat. Neonatol. Nurs. 2:11-19.
30. Cordero, L., and F.P. Zuspan. 1988. Very low-birth weight infants: five years experience of a regional perinatal program. Ohio Med. 84:976-978.
31. Hanau-Walsh, J. 1982. Evaluating the effectiveness of a perinatal outreach education program. J. Obstet. Gynecol. Neonatal Nurs. 11:226-229.
32. Handler, A., D. Rosenberg, M. Driscoll, M. Cohen, E. Swift, P. Garcia, and J. Cohn. 1991. Regional perinatal care in crisis: a case study of an urban public hospital. J. Public Health Pol. 12:184-198.
33. Harness, B. 1989. The benefits of cooperation in perinatal health care. Trustee 42:19, 27.
34. Hulsey, T.C., H.C. Heins, T.A. Marshall, M.L. Martin, T.W. McGee, M.C. Meglen, S.F. Peden, W.B. Pittard, and D.H. Wells. 1989. Regionalized perinatal care in South Carolina. J. S. C. Med. Assoc. 85:357-384.
35. Borker, S., C. Rudolph, T. Tsuruki, and M. Williams. 1990. Interhospital referral of high-risk newborns in a rural regional perinatal program. J. Perinatol. 10:156-163.
36. Gagnon, D., S. Allison-Cooke, and R.M. Schwartz. 1988. Perinatal care: the threat of deregionalization. Pediatr. Ann. 17:447-452.
37. Grassi, L.C. 1988. Life, money, quality: the impact of regionalization on perinatal/neonatal intensive care. Neonatal Netw. 6:53-59.
38. Kanto, W.P., Jr. 1987. Regionalization revisited (editorial). Am. J. Dis. Child. 141:403-404.
39. Caldwell, M. 1991. Financing nutrition programs. Pp. 289-302 in C. Sharbaugh, ed. Call to Action: Better Nutrition for Mothers, Children, and Families. National Center for Education in Maternal and Child Health, Washington, D.C.
40. Hill, I.T., and T. Bennett. 1990. Enhancing the Scope of Prenatal Services. National Governors' Association, Washington, D.C.
41. Schleuning, D., G. Rice, and R.A. Rosenblatt. 1991. Addressing barriers to perinatal care: a case study of the Access to Maternity Care Committee in Washington State. Public Health Rep. 106:47-52.
42. Stephens, D., E. Dennis, M. Toomer, and J. Holloway. 1991. The diversity of case management needs for the care of homeless persons. Public Health Rep. 106:15-19.
43. Wiecha, J.L., J.T. Dwyer, and M. Dunn-Strohecker. 1991. Nutrition and health services needs among the homeless. Public Health Rep. 106:364-374.
44. Institute of Medicine. 1992. Nutrition During Pregnancy and Lactation: An Implementation Guide. Report of the Subcommittee for a Clinical Applications Guide, Committee on Nutritional Status During Pregnancy and Lactation, Food and Nutrition Board. National Academy Press, Washington, D.C.

2

Nutritional Concerns of Women in the Preconceptional, Prenatal, and Postpartum Periods

This chapter reviews key aspects of maternal nutrition in three periods—before conception, during pregnancy, and after delivery—and identifies health conditions that call for special nutrition services during those periods. Because breastfeeding increases the need for postpartum nutrition services, breastfeeding women are distinguished from non-breastfeeding women.

PRECONCEPTIONAL NUTRITION

As noted in *Caring for Our Future: The Content of Prenatal Care*, "the preconception visit may be the single most important health care visit when viewed in the context of its effect on pregnancy" (p. 26).[1]

Goals of Preconceptional Nutrition Services

Preconception visits[a] provide valuable opportunities to reduce women's exposure to risk factors that influence their nutritional status and thus to improve their overall nutritional status before conception. This, in turn,

---

[a]The term preconception visits may be applied to periodic health visits for women, to family planning visits, or to visits specifically targeted to preparing for conception.

may decrease the likelihood of unfavorable pregnancy outcomes, such as the delivery of a premature or low-birth-weight infant. Several sources agree that nutritional services should be one of several components of preconceptional care.[1-4] The publications *ACOG Guide to Planning for Pregnancy, Birth, and Beyond*[5] and *Caring for Our Future: The Content of Prenatal Care*[1] list nutrition-related topics to address at a preconception visit.

An increased emphasis on preconceptional care acknowledges that achieving substantial changes in diet and lifestyle often involves making incremental changes over time. It also recognizes that the primary prevention of nutrition-related fetal malformations or spontaneous abortions is possible only if risk reduction activities begin before conception; even an early prenatal visit would ordinarily be too late for effective intervention. Addressing behavioral change before conception can allow a woman to identify constructive actions and to delay conception until she has achieved a healthier physical state—one that will increase her chances for a successful pregnancy outcome.

Providing nutritional assessment, education, and interventions to encourage an optimal state of health may also benefit the many women who do not desire pregnancy. For these women, the provision of nutritional care as part of a periodic health assessment can be a mechanism for promoting their health over the short term, with the potential for preventing problems in the event of an unplanned pregnancy and for preventing or retarding the development of chronic diseases later in life.[6]

The objectives of nutritional care in the preconceptional period are to encourage women to achieve appropriate weight for height and healthful dietary habits. To this end, a periodic health visit for women of childbearing age should include assessment to identify indicators of possible nutrition problems, education relating to healthful dietary practices, and counseling, referral, or other interventions as needed to solve or reduce the adverse effects of such problems. Detailed information on these care activities is given in *Nutrition During Pregnancy and Lactation: An Implementation Guide*.[7]

The following section briefly discusses the nutrition-related health conditions that have been most closely linked to unfavorable pregnancy outcomes. There are also other health conditions occurring prior to conception that may increase the risk of nutrition problems during pregnancy, but data on such relationships are sparse. Data are also lacking on the relationship of multiple socioeconomic problems prior to conception and the risk of nutrition-related difficulties during pregnancy.

Health Conditions Warranting Special Nutrition Services Before Pregnancy

Exposure of a woman to either excessive or inadequate amounts of certain nutrients early in the first trimester of pregnancy may lead to spontaneous abortion or congenital malformations. Exposure to high, potentially harmful amounts of a nutrient is possible under several circumstances: if the woman has a metabolic condition (such as diabetes mellitus or phenylketonuria) that causes excessive maternal blood levels of one or more nutrients; if the mother takes high doses of retinol (preformed vitamin A); or if she takes a potentially teratogenic medication such as isotretinoin (a vitamin A analogue). Very low nutrient levels are possible if the mother's diet is chronically inadequate or if she takes certain medications or other substances that alter her metabolism or deplete her nutritional stores. For example, the medicines methotrexate and diphenylhydantoin (Dilantin®) alter folate metabolism, and alcohol increases the urinary excretion of zinc. For more information on these topics, see, for example, Berkowitz and colleagues,[8] Briggs and others,[9] the 1990 Institute of Medicine report *Nutrition During Pregnancy*,[10] and Niebyl.[11]

Preexisting Diabetes Mellitus

Women whose pregnancies are complicated by preexisting diabetes mellitus are at increased risk for delivering infants with major congenital malformations.[12] These malformations occur in the first weeks after conception, often well before many women enter prenatal care. Many of these anomalies, however, may be prevented by the normalization of maternal blood glucose values throughout the first 12 weeks of gestation.[13] For blood glucose values to be normal at conception, it is desirable to provide the nutrition and medical services needed to achieve metabolic control well *before* conception.[14,15] In one recent study that involved intensive education and treatment, the incidence of major congenital anomalies in the group treated before conception was 1.2%, compared with 10.9% in the group treated at 6 weeks of gestation or later.[16] Scheffler and colleagues[17] reported that early enrollment (before 8 weeks' gestation) in the California Diabetes and Pregnancy Program, which has a strong nutrition component, had a high cost-benefit ratio: for each $1 spent on the program, the estimated short-term savings exceeded $5.

Phenylketonuria

Phenylketonuria (PKU) is an inherited condition involving the inability to metabolize phenylalanine, an essential amino acid. Until recently, treatment to control serum levels of phenylalanine[18] had been targeted mainly to infants and children: if treatment with a phenylalanine-restricted diet is initiated early in infancy, it helps prevent abnormal brain development and severe mental retardation while allowing normal growth. This rather complicated diet (which requires the use of expensive, specially formulated low-phenylalanine products) is usually discontinued in adulthood, when elevated serum levels of phenylalanine have been presumed to be no longer neurotoxic.

If pregnancy occurs, however, excessive amounts of phenylalanine in the maternal serum are associated with an extremely high incidence of mental retardation, microcephaly, low birth weight, and congenital heart disease among infants who themselves have not inherited PKU.[19-21] There is evidence that the occurrence of these problems can be reduced (although not perhaps eliminated) if the mother maintains a low serum phenylalanine level before conception and throughout pregnancy.[21-24]

To achieve and maintain the desired phenylalanine level, the mother should be identified before pregnancy[25] and helped to modify her intake.[26] For this purpose, she will need intensive support and follow-up by an interdisciplinary team, including a dietitian experienced in the treatment of this disorder. If the mother's intellectual abilities are limited (perhaps because of inadequate dietary control of her condition during her early years), simplified strategies for diet modification and skillful teaching will be needed.[27]

History of Poor Pregnancy Outcome

Two adverse outcomes of a previous pregnancy—neural tube defects (such as spina bifida) and fetal alcohol syndrome—should alert the health care provider to the need for attention to preventive measures before pregnancy.

Once a woman has delivered an infant with a neural tube defect, her risk of delivering another affected infant (often called a recurrent neural tube defect) is very high—2 to 10%.[10] The results of a recent randomized clinical trial in Great Britain[28] indicated that high-dose (4-mg/day) folic acid supplements given before conception and throughout the first trimester were protective against recurrent neural tube defects. (The critical time for the development of the neural tube is 17 to 30 days after conception.) Subsequently, the Centers for Disease Control (CDC)[29] issued specific recommendations for high-dose folic acid supplementation (preconceptionally and throughout the first trimester, under a physician's supervision) to reduce the risk of recurrent neural tube defects. Questions remain concerning the etiology of neural tube defects, the most appropriate dosage, and the appropriate role of nutrition in preventing first occurrences.[30,31]

Previous delivery of an infant with fetal alcohol syndrome calls for efforts to help the mother eliminate or greatly reduce her consumption of alcoholic beverages, if she has not already done so, and to achieve a healthful diet. (See the later section entitled "Conditions Involving Unhealthy Behaviors.")

Extremes of Maternal Weight for Height

The committee found no studies that examined the effects of losing or gaining weight before pregnancy on outcomes of pregnancy. However, because both high and low prepregnancy weight are associated with increased risk of various unfavorable pregnancy outcomes, it is prudent to achieve normal weight for height before conception through healthful diet and exercise. Underweight women are at increased risk of delivering a low-birth-weight infant;[10] they may also be at increased risk of pregnancy complications such as antepartum hemorrhage, premature rupture of the membranes, preterm delivery, anemia, and endometritis.[32,33] Obese women are at increased risk for complications (e.g., chronic hypertension, preeclampsia, gestational diabetes mellitus, and cesarean delivery[34]), and their infants are at increased risk for macrosomia or high birth weight—a condition associated with an increased risk of shoulder dystocia and of maternal and infant morbidity.[10]

If gastric banding or stapling has been used to treat severe obesity, it is advisable to delay conception until metabolic function and dietary intake have stabilized and there has been time to replenish nutrient stores.[35] Both of these types of surgery initially result in greatly reduced food intake; either type can precipitate potentially serious deficiencies of many essential nutrients.

Maternal Eating Disorders

Anorexia nervosa, bulimia, and bulimia nervosa[36,37] are serious eating disorders that affect a small proportion of U.S. women in their childbearing years. Severely restricting food intake may result in general malnutrition (which sometimes is so serious that it prevents ovulation), whereas purging may result in life-threatening fluid and electrolyte imbalances.[38] Women with eating disorders may begin pregnancy in a poor nutritional state; they are at risk of developing imbalances, deficiencies, or weight gain abnormalities during pregnancy if aberrant eating behaviors are not controlled.[39]

Because treatment for these conditions requires long-term psychotherapy and behavior modification, referral for care should be accomplished *before conception* if possible. Published information on this problem during pregnancy is largely anecdotal but suggests that increased efforts are needed to identify women with bulimia nervosa.[40]

Other Chronic Conditions or Diseases

Prior to pregnancy, dietary counseling may substantially improve the nutritional status of women with serious chronic gastrointestinal disorders such as Crohn's disease, celiac disease, or liver disorders. Preconceptional nutritional interventions such as weight loss programs for the treatment of hypertension and modified diets to control blood lipids may be useful alternatives to medications that are not considered desirable for the fetus.

PRENATAL NUTRITION

Nutrition exerts an important influence on pregnancy outcome.[10,41] The U.S. surgeon general,[41] the publication *Healthy People 2000*,[42] and many expert groups (e.g., the American Academy of Pediatrics and the American College of Obstetricians and Gynecologists,[2] the American Nurses Association,[43] the Public Health Service Expert Panel on the Content of Prenatal Care,[1] the Institute of Medicine,[44] and the U.S. Preventive Services Task Force[45]) have all pointed out the value of interventions to help pregnant women achieve adequate diets. Congress has tangibly recognized the importance of prenatal nutrition by appropriating funds for the Special Supplemental Food Program for Women, Infants, and Children (WIC) continuously since 1974 (see Chapter 1). Moreover, at least 18 states have appropriated state funds to extend the reach of the WIC program (B. Jendrysik, Food and Nutrition Service, U.S. Department of Agriculture, personal communication, 1991).

Nutritional Demands of Normal Pregnancy

During pregnancy, maternal requirements for all nutrients increase; this is reflected in higher Recommended Dietary Allowances (RDAs)[46] for most nutrients during pregnancy (see Table 2-1). For some nutrients, the evidence indicates a direct link between chronic maternal deficiencies and poor outcomes for the mother or the infant. For example, prolonged deficiency of iron, folate, or vitamin B_{12} (or any combination of these) may lead to anemia in the mother; deficiency of vitamin D may lead to neonatal hypocalcemia and to maternal osteomalacia; and deficiency of vitamin A may lead to restricted fetal growth.[10] On the other hand, excessive intake of some nutrients may be harmful to the fetus, especially very early in pregnancy (see the previous section, "Preconceptional Nutrition").

In addition, total food intake (which serves as a proxy for energy intake) influences gestational weight gain. A large body of evidence indicates that gestational weight gain, particularly during the second and third trimesters, is an important determinant of fetal growth. Table 2-2 summarizes recommendations for total gestational weight gain. In a study of nearly 7,000 births, Parker and Abrams[47] found that maternal weight gains within these recommended ranges were associated with better outcomes: fewer infants were either small for gestational age or large for gestational age, and fewer woman had cesarean deliveries.

Nutrients

A well-balanced diet is the appropriate source of nutrients during pregnancy. For the majority of pregnant women, iron is the only nutrient for which requirements cannot reasonably be met by diet alone. The 1990 IOM report *Nutrition During Pregnancy*[10] recommends a daily supplement containing 30 mg of ferrous iron as a part of routine care during the second and third trimesters; the report also recommends that guidance be provided for the safe, effective use of this supplement. Routine determination of the hemoglobin value or hematocrit is advised to identify women who need higher iron intake.

TABLE 2-1 Recommended Dietary Allowances for Nonpregnant, Pregnant, and Lactating Women[a]

Nutrient and Units	Nonpregnant[b] 15–24 yrs	Nonpregnant[b] ≥25 yrs	Pregnant[c]	Lactating[c] 1st 6 mos	Lactating[c] 2nd 6 mos
Energy (kcal)	2,200	2,200	2,500	2,700	2,700
Protein (g)	44–46	50	60	65	62
Vitamin A (μg RE)	800	800	800	1,300	1,200
Vitamin D (μg)	10	5	10	10	10
Vitamin E (mg α-TE)	8	8	10	12	11
Vitamin C (mg)	60	60	70	95	90
Thiamin (mg)	1.1	1.1	1.5	1.6	1.6
Riboflavin (mg)	1.3	1.3	1.6	1.8	1.7
Niacin (mg NE)	15	15	17	20	20
Vitamin B_6 (mg)	1.5	1.6	2.2	2.1	2.1
Folacin (μg)	180	180	400	280	260
Vitamin B_{12} (μg)	2.0	2.0	2.2	2.6	2.6
Calcium (mg)	1,200	800	1,200	1,200	1,200
Phosphorus (mg)	1,200	800	1,200	1,200	1,200
Magnesium (mg)	280	280	305	355	340
Iron (mg)	15	15	30[d]	15	15
Zinc (mg)	12	12	15	19	16
Iodine (μg)	150	150	175	200	200
Selenium (μg)	55	55	65	75	75

[a]Adapted from the 10th edition of the National Research Council's *Recommended Dietary Allowances*.[46]

[b]This category includes women in the postpartum period if they are not breastfeeding.

[c]Values apply to women of any age.

[d]This intake cannot be met by the iron content of habitual U.S. diets; the daily use of a 30-mg supplement is recommended during the second and third trimesters of pregnancy.

As explained in *Nutrition During Pregnancy,* evidence is not sufficient to warrant routine supplementation of all pregnant women with other nutrients. However, vitamin-mineral supplementation is recommended in certain situations. Therefore, the routine assessment of dietary practices is recommended for all pregnant women in the United States to determine the need for more intensive dietary counseling, for vitamin or mineral supplements, or both. A simple procedure for such assessment is described in *Nutrition During Pregnancy and Lactation: An Implementation Guide.*[7]

TABLE 2-2 Recommended Total Weight Gain Ranges for Pregnant Women[a,b]

Prepregnancy Weight-for-Height Category	Recommended Total Gain	
	lb	kg
Low (BMI[c] <19.8)	28–40	12.5–18
Normal (BMI of 19.8 to 26)	25–35	11.5–16
High (BMI >26.0 to 29.0)	15–25	7.0–11.5
Obese (BMI >29.0)	≥15	≥7.0

[a]Adapted from the Institute of Medicine's *Nutrition During Pregnancy.*[10]

[b]For singleton pregnancies. The range for women carrying twins is 35 to 45 lb (16 to 20 kg). Young adolescents (<2 years after menarche) and African-American women should strive for gains at the upper end of the range. Short women (<62 in, or <157 cm) should strive for gains at the lower end of the range.

[c]BMI = body mass index.

The dispensing of supplements, however, is not considered a satisfactory substitute for a well-balanced diet or for taking steps to improve access to food.[10]

Energy

Pregnant women need a sufficient intake of energy to support recommended weight gain. "Women who are thinner before pregnancy tend to have babies that are smaller than those of their heavier counterparts with the *same* gestational weight gain" (p. 8).[10] Thus, women who enter pregnancy with low weight for height may need to devote extra attention to achieving adequate weight gain to reduce their risk of delivering low-birth-weight babies.

Screening for factors that may interfere with adequate weight gain is recommended for all pregnant women, as is the monitoring of weight gain over the course of pregnancy.

Nutrition in Complicated Pregnancies

The combination of pregnancy and a health problem often leads to complex nutritional problems that require the attention of a specialized team. For example, pregnancy makes it more important (and more difficult) to control the blood glucose of a woman with diabetes mellitus. On the other hand, some conditions that complicate pregnancy, such as multiple gestation and chronic hypertension, ordinarily require increased attention to basic nutrition services but not complex dietary management.

The following section clarifies why certain conditions ordinarily warrant special nutrition services or extended basic services. The list begins with conditions specific to pregnancy. It then covers various systemic problems, conditions related to unhealthy behaviors, and miscellaneous disorders. Although many of the diseases are quite uncommon, the role of special nutrition services in promoting favorable pregnancy outcomes for some of them is clear. The list of conditions is not all-inclusive: for example, extremely rare conditions such as cystinuria and Wilson's disease are omitted.

Conditions Specific to Pregnancy

Hyperemesis Gravidarum. Severe hyperemesis gravidarum is a serious complication of pregnancy that involves intractable vomiting with dehydration, electrolyte imbalance, ketonuria, weight loss, and possibly neurologic disturbances and liver or renal abnormalities. Death has occurred with severe disease. Conservative therapy includes intravenous hydration, sedation, antiemetic medication, and brief psychotherapy. When these fail to arrest the condition, parenteral nutrition may be life saving.[48,49] In addition to the emotional support and services of a psychotherapist, the advice of a dietitian is often helpful in directing therapy; it is invaluable when the woman is fed parenterally.

Increased Risk for Preterm Birth. In the United States, approximately 7% of newborn babies are of low birth weight (that is, they weigh less than 2,500 g),[42] and in the majority of cases, the cause is preterm delivery.[44] At the first prenatal visit, it is advisable to evaluate all women for the possibility of preterm delivery. Many practitioners use a specific risk score based on a careful history and physical examination to evaluate the potential for this problem (e.g., see Meis et al.[50] and Papiernik et al.[51]). Although there is debate over the accuracy of certain scoring systems, it is well documented that previous preterm birth and certain physical symptoms (uterine cramps, bloody spotting, and increased vaginal mucus discharge) are strong predictors of preterm birth.

There is suggestive evidence that the risk of preterm birth can be reduced by a combination of intensive prenatal visits, uterine activity monitoring, and patient education.[50] So far, studies have not identified which elements of prenatal care are more powerful in preventing preterm birth.

As a part of comprehensive care, women found to be at high risk for preterm birth should be the beneficiaries of intensive evaluation, diet counseling, and, if necessary, food and vitamin-mineral supplementation. Because cigarette smoking, excessive alcohol intake, and illegal substance use all lead to an increased likelihood of preterm birth, the entire health care team needs to assist the woman who uses these substances to quit and to obtain outside help.

If preterm labor occurs and is treated with bedrest and tocolytic therapy, the woman may need extra nutritional care to deal with problems (e.g., decreased appetite, increasing constipation, glucose intolerance) associated with one or both of these treatments.

Multiple Pregnancy. The presence of more than one fetus in a gestation imparts added risk for preterm labor, preeclampsia, and diabetes mellitus. The mother will benefit from nutritional counseling to help her meet her increased nutritional demands comfortably and within any limits that may be imposed on her physical activity. Vitamin-mineral supplementation is advisable in combination with a well-balanced diet.[10] One study[52] indicates that nutritional intervention may reduce the occurrence of low birth weight and of very low birth weight among twins.

Fetal Growth Restriction. The term *fetal growth restriction*, formerly called intrauterine growth retardation, refers to infants born at an abnormally low weight for their gestational age. Among the nutrition-related factors associated with fetal growth restriction are the abuse of many kinds of substances,[53-57] low weight for height, low weight gain during the second and third trimesters,[10] and serious maternal infectious diseases such as acquired immune deficiency syndrome (AIDS). Prenatal participation in WIC (which includes food supplementation and nutrition education) is associated with higher birth weight even among infants born before 37 weeks of gestation.[58] Women who are suspected of having a growth-restricted fetus may need expert and intensive nutritional management.

Systemic Health Problems

Diabetes Mellitus. A primary aim of pregnancy management for the woman with diabetes mellitus is the maintenance of normal blood glucose[59-61] while allowing sufficient energy intake to achieve recommended weight gain. The goal for women with preexisting diabetes mellitus is to achieve normal blood glucose values before conception (see the previous section, "Preconceptional Care") and sustain normal values throughout gestation to minimize the risk for fetal anomalies, fetal death, macrosomia, respiratory distress syndrome, maternal infection, and possibly preeclampsia.[62-65]

The expertise of a dietitian is highly desirable when providing nutrition services for pregnant women with diabetes mellitus. According to the Third International Workshop-Conference on Gestational Diabetes Mellitus (GDM), "nutritional counseling is the cornerstone of the management of all women with GDM. . . ." (p. 200).[61] Nutritional assessment, planning, and counseling are coordinated with medical management as a component of collaborative prenatal care.[17,66-69]

At present, no consensus exists concerning the most favorable dietary recommendations for pregnant women with diabetes mellitus.[69-72] In all approaches, however, the proportion of fat and carbohydrate is controlled in some way, usually the proportion of simple sugars is decreased, and generous intake of food sources of fiber is encouraged. The distribution of food in meals and snacks is also controlled. If insulin is administered, a very careful balance must be struck between diet, physical activity, the insulin dosage, and sometimes other factors (such as infection) that influence metabolism. The self-monitoring of blood glucose with memory-based meters, usually on an outpatient basis, provides useful information for making decisions regarding diet and insulin for the day-to-day maintenance of normal blood glucose.

Hypertensive Disorders. In the past, nutritional interventions such as restriction of energy and sodium were recommended for the prevention of preeclampsia and the treatment of chronic hypertensive disease during pregnancy, but those interventions are no longer recommended.[73,74] The effects of calcium supplementation for women at risk of developing preeclampsia are under study.[10,75,76]

Because pregnancy increases the body's requirement for sodium, sodium restriction is ill-advised. Women who receive medication for hypertensive diseases are now encouraged to avoid excessive intake of salty foods but to salt foods to taste. Diuretics are seldom required except in the presence of cardiopulmonary failure or in the rare case of resistance to other forms of antihypertensive therapy.

Renal Disorders. Advanced renal disease and chronic renal failure are conditions rarely seen among pregnant women. Nonetheless, women with these conditions require special nutrition services (see, for example, Fröhling and colleagues[77]) to balance the increased nutrient requirements of pregnancy, the impaired ability to excrete certain nutrients, and the increased losses of certain nutrients that may result from dialysis or drug treatment. Close monitoring is critically important to guide dietary adjustments.

Human Immunodeficiency Virus. Because women infected with human immunodeficiency virus (HIV) are at increased risk for problems with gastrointestinal function, weight loss, and anemia,[78,79] it is prudent to provide a thorough initial nutritional assessment, to recommend vitamin-mineral supplementation, and to monitor the woman's nutritional status frequently. This is especially important for women with AIDS. Because the effect of the virus on the fetus appears to be quite varied and unpredictable, it seems advisable to provide dietary management that not only avoids maternal weight loss but encourages normal weight gain during pregnancy, provides the nutrients essential to the proper functioning of the immune system,[80] and includes education concerning the prevention of foodborne diseases.[81,82]

Conditions Involving Unhealthy Behaviors

Cigarette Smoking. Maternal cigarette smoking poses a serious threat to both the health and the growth of the developing fetus.[10,83,84] The high frequency of smoking (25 to 30%) among U.S. women[85] makes smoking a national problem as well as an individual one. Women who smoke need strong encouragement to stop this behavior and assistance to do so before and during pregnancy. Attention to the use of smokeless tobacco products is also warranted among some populations (e.g., a substantial proportion of young females from some American Indian tribes use such products;[86,87] S. Pelican, Indian Health Service, personal communication, 1991).

Windsor and colleagues[88] estimate that the dissemination of available, tested, cost-effective smoking cessation methods (with quit rates of 12 to 14%) could lead to cessation by an additional 28,000 pregnant women who are served by the public sector and an additional 84,000 who are served by the private sector each year. Shipp and colleagues[89] present a method for estimating the break-even point for smoking cessation programs for pregnant women.

Pregnancy is a time when all members of the family may be much more willing to try to stop substance abuse of all kinds because of their concern for the fetus, and all members of the family should be offered help. Improved diet and nutritional supplements may help improve fetal outcomes for smokers or former smokers,[90-92] but those measures are not an acceptable substitute for smoking cessation.

Alcohol Use. Alcohol intake during pregnancy—especially if the intake is high—is associated with fetal anomalies, prenatal or postnatal growth restriction, and mental retardation.[93] Information about alcohol abuse often emerges in a nutritional history; all members of the health care team are advised to learn to ask specific questions, such as those presented by Sokol and colleagues,[94] to improve the chance of detecting the problem.[95] Masis and May[96] provide evidence that a comprehensive local program can help to prevent fetal alcohol syndrome. Intensive nutritional management should complement a program of drinking cessation and subsequent support.

Use of Illegal Drugs. Illegal drug use has reemerged as a serious and widespread problem among women of childbearing age in the United States.[10,97] Stimulant drugs such as cocaine and amphetamines are easily obtained. Moreover, the relatively low-cost, highly addictive forms of these drugs, such as "crack" and "ice," are being used with increasing frequency by young men and women. Drug addiction has been associated with serious health problems (including infections such as AIDS, syphilis, and hepatitis); such addiction can also cause serious social and nutritional problems. One major nutritional effect of stimulant drugs is that they suppress the appetite.[98] Moreover, women with limited income may spend all their household food money for drugs or trade their WIC foods and food stamps either for drugs or money.

All addicted women, no matter what drug or drugs they are using, need comprehensive, concentrated nutritional assistance and counseling to complement their prenatal care and drug rehabilitation programs.

Miscellaneous Disorders

Phenylketonuria. Pregnancy complicated by PKU is rare, but the consequences of inadequate dietary treatment are serious and potentially quite costly. Dietary treatment prior to conception (see "Preconceptional Nutrition") and throughout gestation may help to reduce the high rates of spontaneous abortion, mental retardation, microcephaly, and congenital heart disease seen in the offspring of these pregnancies.[20,27] Because of changing protein and energy needs over the course of pregnancy, frequent, careful monitoring and evaluation are advisable to determine the need for dietary adjustments. Some women may need assistance to be able to obtain the expensive formula that is the foundation of the diet.

Gastrointestinal Disorders. The pregnant woman with preexisting primary disease of the gallbladder, pancreas, stomach, or intestine (including malabsorption syndrome and conditions that have led to extensive resection of the intestine) is likely to benefit from special nutrition services to promote optimal maternal and fetal outcomes, as will women with other conditions that interfere with food intake by mouth (e.g., see Granström and colleagues[99]). Special formulas, tube feeding, or parenteral nutrition may be required to provide sufficient nutrients to support both the mother and fetus. If the gastrointestinal tract can be used, many types of tube feeding mixtures and delivery methods can be considered. The type of feeding and the volume of it to be delivered must be individualized for the pregnant woman's needs.

Parenteral feedings generally contain a nonprotein energy source (glucose, fat emulsions, or both), amino acids, electrolytes (including calcium, magnesium, and phosphorus), trace elements, and both water- and fat-soluble vitamins in amounts individualized to the woman's needs. Total parenteral nutrition has been reported to reverse gestational weight loss and to promote fetal growth.[100] This highly specialized feeding method may be used for a relatively brief or extended period either in the hospital or at home, during any trimester of pregnancy.[101-105] Watson and colleagues[106] support the use of peripheral as well as central routes of administration. Close monitoring of the patient and adjustment of the feeding regimen as needed are essential when alternative feeding methods must be used. Extensive training is required for home use of such methods. (See also Chart 3-3, Chapter 3.)

Cystic Fibrosis. Nutritional care for women with cystic fibrosis includes the use of pancreatic enzymes (in pancreatic-insufficient patients); a high-energy, nutrient-rich diet; and supplemental vitamins. Because women with cystic fibrosis may have difficulty consuming and absorbing enough nutrients, they are at increased risk of low weight gain during pregnancy.[107] They may need extra nutritional support using alternative feeding methods such as parenteral nutrition,[108] especially if the work of breathing interferes with adequate dietary intake. Glucose intolerance may occur, further complicating nutritional management.

Other. Cancer, cerebral palsy, and many other conditions may greatly complicate the nutritional care of pregnant women if they interfere with adequate food intake by mouth.

POSTPARTUM NUTRITION

Basic nutrition services for all women warrant increased attention during the postpartum period, but nutritional requirements and the kinds of nutrition services needed at this time differ, depending on whether or not the woman is breastfeeding. The main nutritional focus may be on efforts to replenish nutrient stores, achieve adequate nutrient intake during lactation, or assist with breastfeeding (see Chapter 4). Regardless of breastfeeding status, many women are concerned about returning to their prepregnancy weight and are likely to need guidance to do so in a way that promotes their health.

A study by Caan and colleagues[109] indicates that interconceptional dietary intervention may improve the outcome of a subsequent pregnancy. Women with intervals of ≤ 27 months between pregnancies, who did not breastfeed but who received benefits from WIC during the first 5 to 7 months of the postpartum period, had heavier, longer infants in their second pregnancy than did women who received WIC benefits for 2 months or less post partum. This difference occurred even though both groups of women had received WIC benefits during pregnancy. On average, infants born to the women who were supplemented for 5 to 7 months postpartum weighed 131 g more, were 0.3 cm longer, and had a lower risk of being of low birth weight.

Replenishing Nutrient Stores

Stores of several nutrients (e.g., calcium, vitamin B_6, folate) may need to be replenished during the postpartum period. Women who do not consume an adequate diet despite counseling, or those who are in high-risk categories because of having carried more than one fetus or because of heavy smoking, alcohol abuse, or abuse of illegal drugs,[10] may benefit from continuing to take the low-dose multivitamin-mineral supplement that was prescribed during pregnancy.

Dietary iron requirements during the postpartum period decrease to nonpregnant levels unless blood loss exceeded the usual amount lost during a vaginal delivery (approximately 500 ml).[110] Hemoglobin and hematocrit values ordinarily rise post partum with the contraction of blood volume to nonpregnant levels. In addition, the gradual disintegration of excess red blood cells releases iron that can be used for the synthesis of new hemoglobin.

Nutrition Recommendations for Lactating Women

Diet and Lactation in General

As described in *Nutrition During Lactation*,[111] lactation is a robust process. Milk quantity and quality are maintained reasonably well within a wide range of maternal diets, presumably reflecting subsidy of lactation by maternal stores.

The RDAs for most nutrients are increased during lactation (see Table 2-1)—in some cases by more than 50%.[46] The extra nutrient intake needed to cover exclusive breastfeeding for 4 to 6 months is substantially greater than that needed to cover the entire pregnancy. It is appropriate to encourage intake of a wide assortment of nutritious foods during lactation to help meet a woman's increased nutrient needs.

Specific Nutrients and Energy

During lactation, the nutrients that are most likely to be consumed in lower than recommended amounts are calcium, magnesium, zinc, vitamin B_6, and folate.[111] In general, an additional 500 kcal of energy daily is recommended throughout lactation.[46] This recommendation assumes that there will be gradual loss of maternal body fat to supply some of the energy needed during lactation. A higher increment in energy intake is recommended for lactating women who are slender. Higher energy intake is also needed by women who produce unusually large amounts of milk (for example, those who nurse more than one infant or who donate to a milk bank) and by women who are very active physically (such as those who participate in more than 45 minutes of aerobic exercise daily).

Diet for and Supplementation of the Lactating Woman

The increased needs for nutrients of a lactating woman can be provided by a well-balanced diet.[111] *Nutrition During Pregnancy and Lactation: An Implementation Guide*[7] outlines appropriate dietary guidance for healthy lactating women. For women enrolled in WIC, the program provides food supplements that help supply the extra nutrients needed during lactation.

Among apparently healthy lactating women, situations that may justify nutrient supplementation can be identified by a brief screening process.[111] However, measures to improve dietary intake of nutrients are strongly preferred over supplementation with pharmaceutical preparations,[111] especially since lactation substantially increases the demand for energy, protein, and minerals such as calcium. Multivitamin-mineral supplements do not provide energy or protein, and they provide little calcium.

Weight Loss

From the standpoint of the patient, return to prepregnancy body weight appears to be one of the most common postpartum nutritional concerns. Women who need or want assistance with weight loss can be helped with information about expected weight changes: many women will gain weight during the first 4 days after delivery, but by the fifth postpartum day, most will have begun to lose weight.[112] An above-average rate of weight loss immediately post partum occurs among women who experienced hypertension or preeclampsia during pregnancy—probably because of postpartum diuresis.[113] Women ordinarily lose weight through 4 to 6 months post partum;[114] however, some women gain weight, even if they are breastfeeding. After a period of rapid weight loss in the first few weeks post partum, the average rate of weight loss by lactating women is 0.5 to 1.0 kg (~1 to 2 lb) per month through the sixth month post partum.[111]

If weight loss is an appropriate goal, the woman should be encouraged to set a reasonable body weight goal, and she should be assisted in developing a healthful plan for achieving that goal. For overweight breastfeeding women, the maximum suggested rate of weight loss after the first month post partum is about 2 kg (~4.5 lb)/month.[111] The total energy intake by these women should not be less than 1,800 kcal/day to allow adequate intakes of protein, vitamins, and minerals. Although this level of energy intake may seem high to some women who are familiar with reducing diets, it takes into account the energy required for breastfeeding. Liquid diets and weight loss medications are not recommended.

Conditions Warranting Special Nutrition Services

Most women have no need for special nutrition services immediately after delivery. Those who have delivered by cesarean section may require temporary diet modifications that consider the effects of the surgery and anesthesia on their gastrointestinal function. Women with chronic disorders that call for modified diets require postpartum modifications to adjust for their changing physiologic status and nutrient needs, especially if they are breastfeeding. For example, breastfeeding women who require insulin are at increased risk for hypoglycemia and thus need adequate monitoring and diet counseling.[115]

Special Considerations at the Postpartum Visit

The postpartum visit (usually 4 to 6 weeks following delivery) offers an opportunity to address new or continuing nutritional problems or breastfeeding concerns (see Chapter 4 for information about breastfeeding support). Many women experience some emotional lability (especially symptoms of mild depression) during the postpartum period; some families find it difficult to adapt to the newborn; and families with twins or multiple offspring are confronted with special challenges. Consequently, it is advisable for the primary care provider to determine whether any such stresses are present and whether they are adversely affecting the mother's appetite, access to food, and sleeping or eating habits. In addition, it is recommended that care be taken to identify cases of substance abuse or addiction (including cigarette smoking, alcohol consumption, or illicit use of other mood-altering drugs).

The health status of women who experienced complications during pregnancy should be reassessed at the postpartum visit. For example, assessment of blood glucose status is appropriate for women who experienced gestational diabetes, assessment of blood pressure and of renal status may be indicated for women who experienced preeclampsia, and monitoring of iron status is desirable for women at increased risk of anemia because of hemorrhage associated with delivery. If any abnormal findings are observed, special nutrition services may be initiated.

The postpartum visit also offers an opportunity to promote healthful eating for the entire family and to verify that the infant is receiving well baby care. Information can be provided about meal planning, food preparation, and nutritious food choices for children in the household as well as for adults. A diet rich in grains and cereals, fruits and vegetables, and low-fat dairy products and meats is as appropriate for children over 2 years of age as it is for adults.

SUMMARY

Beginning before conception and extending throughout pregnancy and lactation, primary care providers need to integrate basic nutrition services into their care and to be on the alert for conditions that call for special nutrition services.

REFERENCES

1. Department of Health and Human Services. 1989. Caring for Our Future: The Content of Prenatal Care. A Report of the Public Health Service Expert Panel on the Content of Prenatal Care. Public Health Service, Washington, D.C.
2. American Academy of Pediatrics/American College of Obstetricians and Gynecologists. 1992. Guidelines for Perinatal Care, 3rd ed. American Academy of Pediatrics, Elk Grove, Ill.
3. Harrison, E.A. 1990. Preconception and postconception care of women with medical illness. Pp. 89-108 in I.R. Merkatz and J.E. Thompson, eds. New Perspectives on Prenatal Care. Elsevier, New York.
4. Jack, B., and L. Culpepper. 1990. Preconception care. Pp. 69-88 in I.R. Merkatz and J.E. Thompson, eds. New Perspectives on Prenatal Care. Elsevier, New York.
5. American College of Obstetricians and Gynecologists. 1990. ACOG Guide to Planning for Pregnancy, Birth, and Beyond. American College of Obstetricians and Gynecologists, Washington, D.C.
6. National Research Council. 1989. Diet and Health: Implications for Reducing Chronic Disease Risk. Report of the Committee on Diet and Health, Food and Nutrition Board, Commission on Life Sciences. National Academy Press, Washington, D.C.
7. Institute of Medicine. 1992. Nutrition During Pregnancy and Lactation: An Implementation Guide. Report of the Subcommittee for a Clinical Applications Guide, Committee on Nutritional Status During Pregnancy and Lactation, Food and Nutrition Board. National Academy Press, Washington, D.C.
8. Berkowitz, R., D. Coustan, and T. Mochizuki. 1986. Handbook for Prescribing Medications During Pregnancy. Little, Brown, and Co., Boston.
9. Briggs, G.G., R.K. Freeman, and S.J. Yaffe. 1990. Drugs in Pregnancy and Lactation, 3rd ed. Williams and Wilkins, Baltimore.
10. Institute of Medicine. 1990. Nutrition During Pregnancy: Weight Gain and Nutrient Supplements. Report of the Subcommittee on Nutritional Status and Weight Gain During Pregnancy and the Subcommittee on Dietary Intake and Nutrient Supplements

During Pregnancy, Committee on Nutritional Status During Pregnancy and Lactation, Food and Nutrition Board. National Academy Press, Washington, D.C.

11. Niebyl, J.R., ed. 1988. Drug Use in Pregnancy, 2nd ed. Lea & Febiger, Philadelphia.
12. Becerra, J.E., M.J. Khoury, J.F. Cordero, and J.D. Erickson. 1990. Diabetes mellitus during pregnancy and the risks for specific birth defects a population-based case-control study. Pediatrics 85:1-9.
13. Langer, O. 1990. Critical issues in diabetes and pregnancy: early identification, metabolic control, and prevention of adverse outcome. Pp. 445-460 in I.R. Merkatz and J.E. Thompson, eds. New Perspectives on Prenatal Care. Elsevier, New York.
14. Centers for Disease Control. 1986. Public health guidelines for enhancing diabetes control through maternal- and child-health programs. Morbid. Mortal. Wkly. Rep. 35:201-213.
15. Hollingsworth, D.R., O.W. Jones, and R. Resnick. 1984. Expanded care in obstetrics for the 1980s: preconception and early postconception counseling. Am. J. Obstet. Gynecol. 149:811-814.
16. Kitzmiller, J.L., L.A. Gavin, G.D. Gin, L. Jovanovic-Peterson, E.K. Main, and W.D. Zigrang. 1991. Preconception care of diabetes. Glycemic control prevents congenital anomalies. J. Am. Med. Assoc. 265:731-736.
17. Scheffler, R.M., L.B. Feuchtbaum, and C.S. Phibbs. 1992. Prevention: the cost-effectiveness of the California Diabetes and Pregnancy Program. Am. J. Public Health 82:168-175.
18. Schuett, V.E., and E.S. Brown. 1984. Diet policies of PKU clinics in the United States. Am. J. Public Health 74:501-503.
19. Dimperio, D. 1990. Preconceptional nutrition. J. Pediatr. Perinatal Nutr. 2:65-78.
20. Drogari, E., I. Smith, M. Beasley, and J.K. Lloyd. 1987. Timing of strict diet in relation to fetal damage in maternal phenylketonuria. Lancet 2:927-930.
21. Trahms, C.M. 1989. Maternal hyperphenylalaninemia. Pp. 193-199 in B.S. Worthington-Roberts and S.R. Williams, eds. Nutrition in Pregnancy and Lactation, 4th ed. Times Mirror/Mosby, St. Louis.
22. Koch, R., E. Wenz, C. Bauman, E.G. Friedman, C. Azen, K. Fishler, and W. Heiter. 1988. Treatment outcome of maternal phenylketonuria. Acta Paediatr. Jpn. 30:410-416.
23. Lenke, R.R., and H. L. Levy. 1980. Maternal phenylketonuria and hyperphenylalaninemia. An international survey of the outcome of untreated and treated pregnancies. N. Engl. J. Med. 303:1202-1208.
24. Lynch, B.C., D.B. Pitt, T.G. Maddison, J.E. Wraith, and D.M. Danks. 1988. Maternal phenylketonuria: successful outcome in four pregnancies treated prior to conception. Eur. J. Pediatr. 148:72-75.
25. Waisbren, S.E., L.B. Doherty, I.V. Bailey, F.J. Rohr, and H.L. Levy. 1988. The New England Maternal PKU Project: identification of at-risk women. Am. J. Public Health 78:789-792.
26. American Academy of Pediatrics, Committee on Genetics. 1991. Maternal phenylketonuria. Pediatrics 88:1284-1285.
27. Davidson, D.C. 1989. Maternal phenylketonuria. Postgrad. Med. J. 65 (suppl. 2):S10-S20.
28. MRC Vitamin Study Research Group. 1991. Prevention of neural tube defects: results of the Medical Research Council Vitamin Study. Lancet 338:131-137.
29. Centers for Disease Control. 1991. Use of folic acid for prevention of spina bifida and other neural tube defects–1983–1991. Morbid. Mortal. Wkly. Rep. 40:513-516.
30. Lancet. 1991. Folic acid and neural tube defects (editorial). Lancet 338:153-154.

31. Willett, W.C. 1992. Folic acid and neural tube defect: can't we come to closure? (commentary). Am. J. Publ. Health 82:666-668.
32. Edwards, L.E., I.R. Alton, M.I. Barrada, and E.Y. Hakanson. 1979. Pregnancy in the underweight woman. Course, outcome, and growth patterns of the infant. Am. J. Obstet. Gynecol. 135:297-302.
33. Schramm, W.F. 1981. Obesity, Leanness and Pregnancy Outcome. Missouri Center for Health Statistics, Jefferson City.
34. Abrams, B., and J. Parker. 1988. Overweight and pregnancy complications. Int. J. Obes. 12:293-303.
35. Richards, D.S., D.K. Miller, and G.N. Goodman. 1987. Pregnancy after gastric bypass for morbid obesity. J. Reprod. Med. 32:172-176.
36. American Psychiatric Association. 1987. Diagnostic and Statistical Manual of Mental Disorders, 3rd ed. American Psychiatric Association, Washington, D.C.
37. Garner, D.M., M.P. Olmstead, and J. Polivy. 1983. Development and validation of a multidimensional eating disorder inventory for anorexia-nervosa and bulimia. Int. J. Eating Disorders 2:15-34.
38. Burke, M.E., and J. Vangellow. 1990. Anorexia nervosa and bulimia nervosa: chronic conditions affecting pregnancy. J. NAACOGS Clin. Issu. Perinat. Women's Health Nurs. 1:240-254.
39. Stewart, D.E., J. Raskin, P.E. Garfinkel, O.L. MacDonald, and G.E. Robinson. 1987. Anorexia nervosa, bulimia, and pregnancy. Am. J. Obstet. Gynecol. 157:1194-1198.
40. Willis, D.C., and C.S. Rand. 1988. Pregnancy in bulimic women. Obstet. Gynecol. 71:708-710.
41. Department of Health and Human Services. 1988. The Surgeon General's Report on Nutrition and Health. DHHS (PHS) Publ. No. 88-50211. Public Health Service. U.S. Government Printing Office, Washington, D.C.
42. Department of Health and Human Services. 1990. Healthy People 2000: National Health Promotion and Disease Prevention Objectives. Public Health Service, Office of the Assistant Secretary for Health, Washington, D.C.
43. American Nurses' Association. 1987. Access to Prenatal Care: Key to Preventing Low Birthweight. American Nurses' Association, Kansas City, Mo.
44. Institute of Medicine. 1985. Preventing Low Birthweight. Report of the Committee to Study the Prevention of Low Birthweight, Division of Health Promotion and Disease Prevention. National Academy Press, Washington, D.C.
45. U.S. Preventive Services Task Force. 1989. Guide to Clinical Preventive Services. Williams & Wilkins, Baltimore, Md.
46. National Research Council. 1989. Recommended Dietary Allowances, 10th ed. Report of the Subcommittee on the Tenth Edition of the RDAs, Food and Nutrition Board, Commission on Life Sciences. National Academy Press, Washington, D.C.
47. Parker, J.D., and B. Abrams. 1992. Prenatal weight gain advice: an examination of the recent prenatal weight gain recommendations of the Institute of Medicine. Am. J. Obstet. Gynecol. 79:664-669.
48. Levine, M.G., and D. Esser. 1988. Total parenteral nutrition for the treatment of severe hyperemesis gravidarum: maternal nutritional effects and fetal outcome. Obstet. Gynecol. 72:102-107.
49. Zibell-Frisk, D., K.-L.C. Jen, and J. Rick. 1990. Use of parenteral nutrition to maintain adequate nutritional status in hyperemesis gravidarum. J. Perinatol. 10:390-395.
50. Meis, P.J., J. M. Ernest, M.L. Moore, R. Michielutte, P.C. Sharp, and P.A. Buescher. 1987. Regional program for prevention of premature birth in northwestern North Carolina. Am. J. Obstet. Gynecol. 157:550-556.

51. Papiernik, E., J. Bouyer, J. Dreyfus, D. Collin, G. Winisdorffer, S. Guegen, M. Lecomte, and P. Lazar. 1985. Prevention of preterm births: a perinatal study in Haguenau, France. Pediatrics 76:154-158.
52. Dubois, S., C. Dougherty, M.-P. Duquette, J.A. Hanley, and J.M. Moutquin. 1991. Twin pregnancy: the impact of the Higgins Nutrition Intervention Program on maternal and neonatal outcomes. Am. J. Clin. Nutr. 53:1397-1403.
53. Dombrowski, M.P., H.M. Wolfe, R.A. Welch, and M.I. Evans. 1991. Cocaine abuse is associated with abruptio placentae and decreased birth weight, but not shorter labor. Obstet. Gynecol. 77:139-141.
54. Hadeed, A.J., and S.R. Siegel. 1989. Maternal cocaine use during pregnancy: effect on the newborn infant. Pediatrics 85:205-210.
55. Hanson, J.W., A.P. Streissguth, and D.W. Smith. 1978. The effects of moderate alcohol consumption during pregnancy on fetal growth and morphogenesis. J. Pediatr. 92:457-460.
56. Petitti, D.B., and C. Coleman. 1990. Cocaine and the risk of low birth weight. Am. J. Public Health 80:25-28.
57. Zuckerman, B., D.A. Frank, R. Hingson, H. Amaro, S.M. Levenson, H. Kayne, S. Parker, R. Vinci, K. Aboagye, L.E. Fried, H. Cabral, R. Timperi, and H. Bauchner. 1989. Effects of maternal marijuana and cocaine use on fetal growth. N. Engl. J. Med. 320:762-768.
58. Devaney, B., L. Bilheimer, and J. Schore. 1990. The Savings in Medicaid Costs for Newborns and Their Mothers from Prenatal Participation in the WIC Program. 281-075/20915. Food and Nutrition Service, Office of Analysis and Evaluation, Department of Agriculture. U.S. Government Printing Office, Washington, D.C.
59. Blumenthal, S.A., and R.W. Abdul-Karim. 1987. Diagnosis, classification, and metabolic management of diabetes in pregnancy: therapeutic impact of self-monitoring of blood glucose and of newer methods of insulin delivery. Obstet. Gynecol. Surv. 42:593-604.
60. Langer, O., J. Levy, L. Brustman, A. Anyaegbunam, R. Merkatz, and M. Divon. 1989. Glycemic control in gestational diabetes mellitus–how tight is tight enough small for gestational age versus large for gestational age? Am. J. Obstet. Gynecol. 161:646-653.
61. Metzger, B.E., and the Organizing Committee. 1991. Summary and recommendations of the Third International Workshop-Conference on Gestational Diabetes Mellitus. Diabetes 40 (suppl. 2):197-201.
62. Fuhrmann, K., H. Reiher, K. Semmler, and E. Glockner. 1984. The effect of intensified conventional insulin therapy before and during pregnancy on the malformation rate in offspring of diabetic mothers. Exp. Clin. Endocrinol. 83:173-177.
63. Lucas, M.J., K.J. Leveno, M.L. Williams, P. Raskin, and P.J. Whalley. 1989. Early pregnancy glycosylated hemoglobin, severity of diabetes, and fetal malformations. Am. J. Obstet. Gynecol. 161:426-431.
64. Miller, E., J.W. Hare, J.P. Cloherty, P.J. Dunn, R.E. Gleason, J.S. Soeldner, and J.L. Kitzmiller. 1981. Elevated maternal hemoglobin A_{1c} in early pregnancy and major congenital anomalies in infants of diabetic mothers. N. Engl. J. Med. 304:1331-1334.
65. Rowe, B.R., C.J. Rowbotham, and A.H. Barnett. 1987. Pre-conception counseling, birth weight, and congenital abnormalities in established and gestational diabetic pregnancy. Diabetes Res. 6:33-35.
66. Anderson, J.W. 1989. Recent advances in carbohydrate nutrition and metabolism in diabetes mellitus. J. Am. Coll. Nutr. 8:61S-67S.
67. Garner, C. 1986. Nutritional care of the pregnant diabetic woman. J. Arkansas Med. Soc. 83:245-250.

68. Knopp, R.H., M.S. Magee, V. Raisys, and T. Benedetti. 1991. Metabolic effects of hypocaloric diets in management of gestational diabetes. Diabetes 40 (suppl. 2):165-171.
69. Jovanovic-Peterson, L., and C.M. Peterson. 1990. Dietary manipulation as a primary treatment strategy for pregnancies complicated by diabetes. J. Am. Coll. Nutr. 9:320-325.
70. Arky, R., J. Wylie-Rosett, and B. El-Beheri. 1982. Examination of current dietary recommendations for individuals with diabetes mellitus. Diabetes Care 5:59-63.
71. Dornhorst, A., J.S.D. Nicholls, F. Probst, C.M. Paterson, K.L. Hollier, R.S. Elkeles, and R.W. Beard. 1991. Calorie restriction for treatment of gestational diabetes. Diabetes 40 (suppl. 2):161-164.
72. Hollingsworth, D.R., and D.M. Ney. 1988. Dietary management of diabetic pregnancy. Pp. 285-311 in A. Reece and D.R. Coustan, eds. Diabetes Mellitus in Pregnancy: Principles and Practice. Churchill Livingstone, New York.
73. Newman, V., and J.T. Fullerton. 1990. Role of nutrition in the prevention of preeclampsia. J. Nurse-Midwifery 35:282-291.
74. Rosso, P. 1990. Nutritional care of gravidas with special problems. Pp. 264-311 in Rosso, P., ed. Nutrition and Metabolism in Pregnancy Mother and Fetus. Oxford University Press, New York.
75. Belizán, J.M., J. Villar, L. Gonzalez, L. Campodonico, and E. Bergel. 1991. Calcium supplementation to prevent hypertensive disorders of pregnancy. N. Engl. J. Med. 325:1399-1405.
76. Marcoux, S., J. Brisson, and J. Fabia. 1991. Calcium intake from dairy products and supplements and the risks of preeclampsia and gestational hypertension. Am. J. Epidemiol. 133:1266-1272.
77. Fröhling, P.T., M. Birnbaum, H. Halle, and K. Lindenau. 1986. Successful pregnancy of a woman with advanced renal failure on nutritional treatment. Nephron 44:195-197.
78. Charny, A., and E.K. Ludman. 1991. Treating malnutrition in AIDS Comparison of dietitians' practices and nutrition care guidelines. J. Am. Diet. Assoc. 91:1273-1274, 1277.
79. Raiten, D.J. 1990. Nutrition and HIV Infection. Life Sciences Research Office, Federation of American Societies for Experimental Biology, Bethesda, Md.
80. Aron, J.M. 1991. Toward rational nutritional support of the human immunodeficiency virus-infected patient. J. Parenter. Enteral Nutr. 15:121-122.
81. Archer, D.L. 1989. Food counseling for persons infected with HIV strategy for defensive living. Public Health Rep. 104:196-198.
82. Filice, G.A., and C. Pomeroy. 1991. Preventing secondary infections among HIV-positive persons. Public Health Rep. 106:503-517.
83. Armstrong, B.G., A.D. McDonald, and M. Sloan. 1992. Cigarette, alcohol, and coffee consumption and spontaneous abortion. Am. J. Public Health 82:85-87.
84. McDonald, A.D., B.G. Armstrong, and M. Sloan. 1992. Cigarette, alcohol, and coffee consumption and prematurity. Am. J. Public Health 82:87-90.
85. Schoenborn, C., and G. Boyd. 1989. Smoking and other tobacco use United States 1987. National Center for Health Statistics: Vital and Health Statistics 10:169.
86. Bruerd, B. 1990. Smokeless tobacco use among Native American school children. Public Health Rep. 105:196-201.
87. Schinke, S.P., R.F. Schilling II, L.D. Gilchrist, M.R. Ashby, and E. Kitajima. 1989. Native youth and smokeless tobacco prevalence rates, gender differences, and descriptive characteristics. Pp. 39-42 in G.M. Boyd and C.A. Darby, eds. Smokeless Tobacco Use in the United States. NCI Monographs. NIH Publ. No. 89-3055. National Cancer Institute, Bethesda, Md.

88. Windsor, R.A., M.E. Dalmat, C.T. Orleans, and E.R. Gritz. 1990. The Handbook to Plan, Implement & Evaluate Smoking Cessation Programs for Pregnant Women. March of Dimes Defects Foundation, White Plains, N.Y.
89. Shipp, M., M.S. Croughhan-Minihane, D.B. Petitti, and A.E. Washington. 1992. Estimation of the break-even point for smoking cessation programs in pregnancy. Am. J. Public Health 82:383-390.
90. Garn, S.M., K. Hoff, and K.D. McCabe. 1979. Is there nutritional mediation of the "smoking effect" on the fetus? Am. J. Clin. Nutr. 32:1181-1187.
91. Metcoff, J., P. Costiloe, W.M. Crosby, S. Dutta, H.H. Sandstead, D. Milne, C.E. Bodwell, and S.H. Majors. 1985. Effect of food supplementation (WIC) during pregnancy on birth weight. Am. J. Clin. Nutr. 41:933-947.
92. Rush, D., Z. Stein, and M. Susser. 1980. A randomized controlled trial of prenatal nutritional supplementation in New York City. Pediatrics 65:683-697.
93. Rosett, H.L. 1980. A clinical perspective of the fetal alcohol syndrome. Alcoholism 4:119-122.
94. Sokol, R.J., S.S. Martier, and J.W. Ager. 1989. The T-ACE questions practical prenatal detection of risk-drinking. Am. J. Obstet. Gynecol. 160:863-870.
95. Beresford, T.P., F.C. Blow, E. Hill, K. Singer, and M.R. Lucey. 1990. Comparison of CAGE questionnaire and computer-assisted laboratory profiles in screening for covert alcoholism. Lancet 336:482-485.
96. Masis, K.B., and P.A. May. 1991. A comprehensive local program for the prevention of fetal alcohol syndrome. Public Health Rep. 106:484-489.
97. Streissguth, A.P., T.M. Grant, H.M. Barr, Z.A. Brown, J.C. Martin, D.E. Mayock, S.L. Ramey, and L. Moore. 1991. Cocaine and the use of alcohol and other drugs during pregnancy. Am. J. Obstet. Gynecol. 164:1239-1243.
98. Mohs, M.E., R.R. Watson, and T. Leonard-Green. 1990. Nutritional effects of marijuana, heroin, cocaine, and nicotine. J. Am. Diet. Assoc. 90:1261-1267.
99. Granström, L., L. Granström, and L. Backman. 1990. Fetal growth retardation after gastric banding. Acta Obstet. Gynecol. Scand. 69:533-536.
100. Kirby, D.F., V. Fiorenza, and R.M. Craig. 1988. Intravenous nutritional support during pregnancy. J. Parenter. Enteral Nutr. 12:72-80.
101. Gatenby, S.J. 1987. Maintenance of pregnancy in Crohn's disease by parenteral nutrition a case study. Human Nutrition Applied Nutrition 41A:345-349.
102. Landon, M.B., S.G. Gabbe, and J.L. Mullen. 1986. Total parenteral nutrition during pregnancy. Clin. Perinat. 13:57-72.
103. Lee, R.V., B.D. Rodgers, C. Young, E. Eddy, and J. Cardinal. 1986. Total parenteral nutrition during pregnancy. Obstet. Gynecol. 68:563-571.
104. Mughal, M.M., J.L. Shaffer, M. Turner, and M.H. Irving. 1987. Nutritional management of pregnancy in patients on home parenteral nutrition. Br. J. Obstet. Gynaecol. 94:44-49.
105. Nugent, F.W., M. Rajala, R.A. O'Shea, P.F. Kolack, M.A. Hobin, M.K. Haimes, and M.L. Ingalls. 1987. Total parenteral nutrition in pregnancy conception to delivery. J. Parenter. Enteral Nutr. 11:424-427.
106. Watson, L.A., A.A. Bommarito, and J.F. Marshall. 1990. Total peripheral parenteral nutrition in pregnancy. J. Parenter. Enteral Nutr. 14:485-489.
107. Canny, G.J., M. Corey, R.A. Livingstone, S. Carpenter, L. Green, and H. Levison. 1991. Pregnancy and cystic fibrosis. Obstet. Gynecol. 77:850-853.
108. Valenzuela, G.J., F.L. Comunale, B.H. Davidson, R.R. Dooley, and T.C.-S. Foster. 1988. Clinical management of patients with cystic fibrosis and pulmonary insufficiency. Am. J. Obstet. Gynecol. 159:1181-1183.

109. Caan, B., D.M. Horgen, S. Margen, J.C. King, and N.P. Jewell. 1987. Benefits associated with WIC supplemental feeding during the interpregnancy interval. Am. J. Clin. Nutr. 45:29-41.

110. Ueland, K. 1976. Maternal cardiovascular dynamics. VII. Intrapartum blood volume changes. Am. J. Obstet. Gynecol. 126:671-677.

111. Institute of Medicine. 1991. Nutrition During Lactation. Report of the Subcommittee on Nutrition During Lactation, Committee on Nutritional Status During Pregnancy and Lactation, Food and Nutrition Board. National Academy Press, Washington, D.C.

112. Greene, G.W., H. Smiciklas-Wright, T.O. Scholl, and R.J. Karp. 1988. Postpartum weight change: how much of the weight gained in pregnancy will be lost after delivery? Obstet. Gynecol. 71:701-707.

113. Dennis, K.J., and W.R. Bytheway. 1965. Changes in body weight after delivery. J. Obstet. Gynaecol. Br. Commonw. 72:94-102.

114. Schauberger, C.W., B.L. Rooney, and L.M. Brimer. 1992. Factors that influence weight loss in the puerperium. Obstet. Gynecol. 79:424-429.

115. Ferris, A.M., C.K. Dalidowitz, C.M. Ingardia, E.A. Reece, F.D. Fumia, R.G. Jensen, and L.H. Allen. 1988. Lactation outcome in insulin-dependent diabetic women. J. Am. Diet. Assoc. 88:317-322.

3

Basic and Special Nutrition Services for Women in the Preconceptional, Prenatal, and Postpartum Periods

Nutrition services are fundamental to the primary health care of women. This chapter covers the delivery of basic nutrition services and of nutrition services for women with conditions requiring special care. It also addresses the personnel and the knowledge and skills necessary to deliver high-quality, patient-centered services.

The maternal and child health unit of the health department in each state offers assistance with standard setting and quality assurance, specialized consultation and technical assistance, inter-agency collaboration, and direct service delivery, as well as with local policies and referral systems for the Special Supplemental Food Program for Women, Infants, and Children (WIC), Medicaid, prenatal care access, perinatology centers for consultation on special conditions, and therapeutic nutrition counseling.

The role of WIC in the provision of nutrition services merits special mention and clarification. WIC can and does play an important role in promoting adequate nutrient intake and in facilitating access to proper prenatal and postpartum health care services. However, WIC is not intended to provide comprehensive nutrition services. Some WIC nutritionists or other "competent professional authorities"[a] do not have the advanced training or experience needed to provide special nutrition services

---

[a]"Competent professional authority," according to federal regulations, is the term applied to "an individual on the staff of the local agency authorized to determine nutritional risk and prescribe supplemental food."[1]

(see "Overview of Special Services" later in this chapter); moreover, the WIC program is not funded at a level sufficient to provide the special nutrition services needed by some high-risk women.

DELIVERY OF BASIC NUTRITION SERVICES

Physicians, midwives, nurse practitioners, and other primary care providers can and should integrate basic nutritional care into the care of all expectant and new mothers. Preconceptional care may be provided as part of a woman's routine health care, in family planning clinics, and during visits specifically to address planning for pregnancy. Excluding delivery, nearly all prenatal care is provided in physicians' or midwives' offices or in prenatal clinics. There is increasing interest, however, in the use of supplemental home visits for high-risk families.[2-5] Most commonly, postpartum care is first provided in the hospital; subsequently, it may be provided in the physician's office or health center, and, in some cases, in the patient's home as well.

Overview of Basic Services

Chart 3-1 lists the nutritional care activities that need to be part of the routine care of all women—regardless of their level of nutritional risk, socioeconomic status, health status, or type of primary care provider. The publication *Nutrition During Pregnancy and Lactation: An Implementation Guide*[6] contains suggestions for integrating these activities into routine care.

Special nutritional care activities for the relatively few women with complex health problems are discussed later in this chapter. If referral to a dietitian or other specialists, or both, is necessary, open lines of communication are essential between the primary care providers and the specialist so that all members of the health care team are in agreement about and reinforce the nutritional advice given to the pregnant woman. Documentation, an important form of communication, appears to need more attention: Peoples-Sheps and colleagues[7] report that although 98% of a large sample of prenatal care records included flow charts for weight, only 38% of them included a separate item for nutritional assessment, 19% an item for nutrition education, and 51% an item for alcohol use.

Personnel

The attending physician, midwife, or nurse should be capable of providing the basic nutritional care measures identified in Chart 3-1. Contacts with a dietitian are encouraged because these health care providers are specially qualified to provide a full range of nutrition services—including the extensive assessment, individualized diet modifications, or other specialized approaches required for a number of nutrition problems. In many instances dietitians are neither members of the obstetrical practice nor on site in the care delivery setting. Thus, it is essential to have a method for identifying women who need special nutrition services and referring them to a dietitian. If referral is not possible because of transportation barriers or other obstacles, alternative methods of consulting with the dietitian should be arranged.

Through in-service or continuing education programs, dietitians can assist health care team members with the basic nutritional care activities listed in Chart 3-1. This is especially important if a dietitian will not be directly involved in the care of women with gestational diabetes mellitus or lactose intolerance. Dietitians can also provide guidance concerning appropriate nutrition education materials for use in waiting rooms, prenatal classes, parenting classes, hospitals (e.g., on closed-circuit television), or other venues.

The effectiveness of nutritional care may be substantially increased by an expanded health care team that provides outreach activities, home visits, and streamlined services, or that uses other strategies to increase the utilization of prenatal care by disadvantaged women.[8] Such activities involve visiting nurses, social workers, dietitians, case managers, trained community health workers, peer counselors, and others.[9]

The support of breastfeeding needs special attention. Because breastfeeding support has not been a standard part of the curriculum for health care providers, the provider who is best qualified in a particular setting is likely to be one who has participated in a program that provides specialized training and guided experience. (For more information about breastfeeding support, see Chapter 4.)

If none of the health care providers in a particular setting is bilingual, trained interpreters should be available by special arrangement to assist with assessment, counseling, and educational activities for patients who are uncomfortable communicating in English. Often, community health workers can be trained to provide this service. With proper training, such workers may also perform a variety of outreach activities and other services for expectant and new mothers (see, e.g., Tindall[10]).

CHART 3-1 Basic Nutritional Care Activities for Expectant and New Mothers

Basic nutritional care activities in support of pregnancy, lactation, and women's health are listed below. They are covered in more detail in Nutrition During Pregnancy and Lactation: An Implementation Guide.[6] *Physicians, physicians' assistants, midwives, nurses, nurse-practitioners, dietitians, and other primary care providers should all participate in integrating these activities into routine care.*

Assessment

- Weigh at each visit; measure height and estimate nonpregnant body mass index at the first visit.
- Monitor and interpret data such as hemoglobin level, blood pressure, and weight change.
- Collect data on attitudes, current dietary practices, cooking facilities, housing, and other factors pertinent to nutritional status.
- Consider the above information to identify women at risk of nutritional problems, that is, those who require more thorough assessment or intervention, or both.

Health Maintenance

- Provide information, education, or counseling concerning the following:
  - diet and fluid intake, weight, managing gastrointestinal discomforts and other common nutrition-related problems, the safe and appropriate use of vitamin-mineral supplements, and avoiding or stopping the use of harmful substances;[a]
  - adjusting dietary intake for relatively common situations such as prescribed bedrest or twin pregnancies;
  - breastfeeding, considering the mother and infant as a unit.
- Recommend a low-dose (30 mg) iron supplement to all pregnant women beginning in the second trimester of pregnancy.[11]

CHART 3-1 *Continued*

Interventions

- Conduct detailed assessments as needed to develop strategies for adjusting nutrient or energy intake or for following up on undesirable changes in weight.
- Provide nutritional counseling for women with commonly occurring conditions such as lactose intolerance, gestational diabetes mellitus controlled by diet and exercise, iron-deficiency anemia, mild gastro-intestinal disorders, obesity, low weight for height, and inadequate prenatal weight gain; or, if possible, refer the woman to a dietitian for this service.
- Recommend nutrient supplements if indicated by the assessment.
- Monitor the woman's progress, and revise the plan of care as indicated.
- Refer the woman, as necessary, to community resources (see Chart 3-2 for federal food and nutrition programs).
- Provide or refer the woman for special nutrition services if she has a health condition that requires complex nutritional care. Such conditions include insulin-requiring diabetes mellitus, certain gastrointestinal diseases, chronic renal failure, and phenylketonuria. For the treatment of eating disorders, the involvement of an experienced eating disorders team is advisable. Follow up on recommendations from nutrition specialists, and confer with them as needed.
- Assist the woman in quitting substance use, or refer her to a special treatment program and follow up as needed.
- Provide special assistance with breastfeeding if the woman wants to breastfeed and has twins, triplets, a premature infant, an infant with a congenital anomaly, or other circumstances that affect feeding or nutrient requirements; or help her obtain this assistance from a lactation specialist.

[a]This includes alerting women to advisories regarding environmental contaminants in the food supply.

CHART 3-2 Eligibility for Federal Food and Nutrition Programs and Program Benefits[a]

Program	Eligibility	Benefits
Special Supplemental Food Program for Women, Infants, and Children (WIC)	Pregnant women, postpartum women (up to 6 months), breastfeeding women (up to 1 year), infants, and children (aged <5 years); must be certified to be at nutritional risk, and household income must be determined to be ≤185%[b] of the federal poverty level[c]	Monthly individualized food packages that include such foods as milk, cheese, eggs, fruit juice, cereal, peanut butter or legumes, infant formula, and infant cereal Nutrition education Referrals
Commodity Supplemental Food Program (CSFP)	Pregnant women, breastfeeding women, other postpartum women, infants, and children (aged <6 years); household income must be determined to be ≤185%[b] of the federal poverty level	Monthly canned or packaged foods including fruits, vegetables, meats, infant formula, farina, beans, other as available
Food Stamp Program	U.S. citizens, recognized refugees with visa status, and legal aliens–all from households with low income and with resources (aside from income) of ≤$2,000 (≤$3,000 with at least one elderly person[d]); eligibility is determined after formal application to local public assistance or social services	Food vouchers, cards, or checks to purchase foods at participating food markets
Temporary Emergency Food Assistance Program (TEFAP)	Households with income ≤150%[b] of the federal poverty level	Quarterly distribution: cheese, butter, rice, occasionally flour, cornmeal, and dry milk. Emergency food available once per month: dairy products, rice, flour, cornmeal
Nutrition Assistance Program (NAP) for Puerto Rico	Residents of Puerto Rico who meet eligibility rules similar to those for the Food Stamp Program	Cash to be used by recipients to supplement their food budget

Food Distribution Program on Indian Reservations (FDPIR)	American-Indian households living on or near reservations	Monthly canned or packaged foods, including fruits, vegetables, meats, beans, grains, flour, cereal, juice, pasta, egg mix, milk, cheese, peanut butter, honey, butter, oil, and shortening
Cooperative Extension–Expanded Food and Nutrition Education Program[e]	Households with children aged <19 years, with income ≤125% of the federal poverty level; at nutritional risk	Education and training regarding food and nutrition

[a]Adapted from Boisvert-Walsh and Kallio, with permission.[9]

[b]Some states have lower cutoff values.

[c]The federal poverty level is computed yearly. The cost of the U.S. Department of Agriculture's Thrifty Food Plan is multiplied by three and adjusted for family size and the current consumer price index.

[d]Elderly are those aged ≥60 years.

[e]This program is not available in all areas.

Knowledge Base and Clinical Skills

A broad base of knowledge and skills (see below) is needed for the delivery of basic nutrition services in support of pregnancy and lactation. Encouraging all health care providers to develop this core of knowledge and skills will facilitate the delivery of consistent, effective nutrition services.

The focus of such knowledge and skills should be on the early identification of complex nutritional problems, treatment and monitoring of patients, and appropriate referrals. More detail can be found in *Nutrition During Pregnancy and Lactation: An Implementation Guide.*[6]

Knowledge and Understanding

- The effects of pregnancy and lactation on recommended nutrient intakes.
- Appropriate ways to increase dietary intake of nutrients.
- Guidelines for nutrient supplementation.
- How restricting the intake of basic food groups affects nutrient intake.
- Recommendations for weight change during pregnancy and lactation and their rationale.
- Principles and techniques of healthful weight management.
- Benefits offered by federally funded food assistance programs for low-income women (see Chart 3-2) and by other community resources, as well as procedures for accessing those resources.
- The techniques of breastfeeding and methods for overcoming common obstacles to successful breastfeeding.
- Basic dietary adjustments for problems that often occur during and after pregnancy.

Assessment Skills

- Accurately measure height and weight.
- Classify women by nonpregnant body mass index.
- Provide basic assessment of dietary practices.
- Interpret information from the patient's history (including diet), laboratory data, and physical examination, and use it to identify women at high risk for nutrition problems before, during, and after pregnancy.

- Monitor and interpret weight changes during pregnancy and post partum.

Health Maintenance Skills

- Provide basic nutrition education about pregnancy and lactation to individuals and groups.
- Assist women to set realistic goals and behavioral objectives targeted toward improving or maintaining their nutritional status.
- Effectively communicate the benefits of breastfeeding, techniques for establishing and maintaining breastfeeding, and strategies for overcoming common obstacles to successful lactation.
- Provide guidance concerning appropriate weight management.
- Educate or counsel women concerning the appropriate use of supplements.

Intervention Skills

- Following established guidelines or protocols, provide basic individualized diet counseling for improving nutrient intake, managing common dietary problems, and addressing inadequate or excessive weight gain.
- Advise on the appropriate use of nutrient supplements for special circumstances.
- Assist the woman to arrange for adequate access to food and other needed resources.
- Arrange for appropriate referral to a dietitian for more thorough assessment and intervention.
- Work with translators, interpreters, or peer counselors as needed for effective care delivery.

Management of the Organization and Delivery of Nutritional Care

- Provide organized in-service education to the health care team (including community outreach workers and peer counselors) concerning the rationale for and the effective delivery of basic nutrition services.
- Participate in evaluation of the overall quality of nutrition services and in identification of appropriate adjustments in care delivery.
- Develop strategies for achieving consistent educational messages and nutritional care practices by various health team members and for triggering appropriate follow-up when there is a change in providers.

DELIVERY OF SPECIAL NUTRITION SERVICES

Certain medical conditions are managed to a large extent by diet modifications or other special forms of nutritional support, and frequent monitoring and revision of the care plan may be needed when the woman is pregnant or lactating. Such conditions usually require specialized nutritional care management by a registered dietitian with experience in pregnancy and lactation as well as in the health problem in question.

High-risk conditions that indicate the need for specific diet therapies include the following:

- hyperemesis gravidarum;
- preexisting diabetes mellitus and gestational diabetes (if insulin is required);
- serious liver or renal disease;
- acquired immune deficiency syndrome (AIDS) or other severe unresponding infection;
- serious gastrointestinal disorders (such as those caused by Crohn's disease or gastric bypass surgery) that lead to inadequate intake or malabsorption;
- genetic disorders that affect nutrition, such as cystic fibrosis and inborn errors of metabolism; and
- serious eating disorders.

Conditions that sometimes entail complicated management include gestational diabetes mellitus treated with diet and exercise, high risk of preterm birth, suspected fetal growth restriction, substance abuse, multifetal gestations, and hypertension. The assessment, planning, and counseling skills of the experienced dietitian may be quite helpful in the care of women with these conditions.

Overview of Special Services

In addition to providing the basic services listed in Chart 3-1, facilities that serve women who have complex nutritional problems should provide the services listed in Chart 3-3.

Treatment of many of the disorders listed in the chart involves frequent calculation of the need for and intake of specific nutrients and development and implementation of an individualized nutritional care plan. The plan should be coordinated with the mother's total care and updated frequently.

Personnel

Highly trained professionals are needed to meet the nutrition challenges posed by pregnancy or lactation complicated by serious health problems. Caring for these women requires a team approach and typically involves a physician, nurse, and dietitian, all of whom have expertise in the care of pregnant and lactating women. For special circumstances, the team will need to be expanded. For example, a physical or occupational therapist may provide necessary services to pregnant or lactating women with certain disabilities, a pharmacist is a valuable addition to a team caring for a pregnant woman who requires parenteral nutrition, and an experienced social worker or public health nurse may help the seriously stressed pregnant woman to marshall the resources she needs for satisfactory management of her condition at home.

The following lists appropriate qualifications for providers of special nutrition services for expectant and new mothers.

- The physician is an obstetrician or a family physician with special training or experience in obstetrics.
- The nurse, nurse-practitioner, and midwife have training and experience in obstetrics.
- The dietitian meets the requirements for registration of the Council for Dietetic Registration and for licensure (where required) and has advanced clinical experience or graduate-level nutrition training that includes extensive clinical experience in prenatal and postpartum care.
- The pharmacist (when needed in support of alternative feeding methods) has an advanced degree in pharmacy or advanced training and supervised experience in nutritional support.
- Outreach workers and peer counselors (when needed to facilitate access to and utilization of care) have completed structured in-service education sessions tailored to local needs and have met the criteria for the program that they will be serving.

CHART 3-3 Special Nutritional Care Activities for Expectant and New Mothers with Complex Needs[a]

- For women who are considering becoming pregnant, provide information on the dietary modifications recommended for the periconceptional period and on the special nutrition-related measures needed to support a healthy pregnancy.
- For women who are attempting to conceive, provide assessment-based dietary counseling.
- Coordinate the nutritional care of pregnant and lactating women who have complex medical or surgical problems.
  - Assess nutritional status.
  - Estimate special nutrient and energy requirements.
  - With the patient (when applicable), plan diet modifications as needed.
  - Develop and implement nutritional care plans in collaboration with others on the health care team. This may include consideration of alternative nutrient delivery methods; use of special food products, nutrient supplements, or enzymes; referral to home health services or to agencies that provide income support or assistance with food and nutrition resources; or any of a wide array of other services that enable the woman to improve her nutritional status.
  - Provide counseling for dietary modifications, and follow up as needed.
  - Instruct other team members (including home visitors, the patient, and the family or significant others, as appropriate) in the special procedures needed to achieve the recommended intakes.
  - Assist with special needs related to breastfeeding (see Chapters 4 and 5).
  - Monitor progress and adjust plans as needed. This may include adapting diet modifications or special feedings over time to respond to the changing needs of the fetus or to the changing milk intake of the breastfed infant.
  - Provide instructional resources for special dietary modifications, and monitor their use.

CHART 3-3 *Continued*

- Collaborate with the eating disorders team as appropriate to promote nutrient intake adequate for a healthy pregnancy and for both maternal and infant needs during breastfeeding.
- Establish effective means of communication to promote consistent, uninterrupted care in inpatient, outpatient, and community settings.

• Provide consultation services for other providers.
• Provide in-service education for health professionals, and help to plan and participate in community education programs.
• Provide leadership in developing activities to monitor and improve the quality and efficiency of the nutrition services being provided.
• Evaluate the results of nutrition interventions for use in program planning.

[a]These activities and services should be available in addition to those listed in Chart 3-1.

Knowledge Base and Clinical Skills

The team that provides nutrition services for women with special nutritional needs must have the knowledge and skills listed earlier for providers of basic nutrition services, as well as the knowledge and skills listed below.

Knowledge and Understanding

• Physiologic and metabolic changes associated with pregnancy and lactation and the diagnostic implications of these changes for high-risk conditions.
• Effects of chronic and acute disease on the course and nutrient requirements of pregnancy and lactation.
• Food-drug-nutrient interactions.
• Principles of diet modification for pregnant and lactating women who have chronic disease or other serious health problems.
• Principles of enteral and parenteral feeding during pregnancy and lactation.

Assessment Skills

- Obtain a comprehensive nutrition history.
- Estimate the woman's nutritional requirements, taking into consideration the effects of health problems and medications on energy balance and nutrient absorption, utilization, and excretion.
- Compare estimated nutrient requirements with nutrient intake from diet, alternative feeding methods, and vitamin-mineral supplements.
- Assess the extent to which social or financial problems must be considered in developing a workable care plan.

Intervention Skills

- Set goals for achievable outcomes, and develop an individualized nutritional care plan to reach those goals, including diet or special feedings, specific behavioral objectives, other interventions, referrals, and monitoring methods and other forms of follow-up.
- Provide nutrition counseling that considers the woman's food habits, changing nutrient requirements, medical or surgical condition, and financial and other constraints and assets. Use counseling strategies suited to the woman's capabilities or those of other primary caretakers at home.
- Monitor the woman's nutritional status and responses to interventions, and recommend changes in the plan of care as indicated.
- Incorporate new knowledge into nutritional care plans and into educational programs for providers.
- Facilitate the family's access to and use of community services, home health, income support, and food and nutrition resources.
- Function effectively within the framework of a multidisciplinary care team.

Management of the Organization and Delivery of Nutritional Care

- Facilitate continuity of nutritional care as the woman moves from the preconceptional period through the prenatal, postpartum, and interconceptional periods—coordinating activities with those of available community services and agencies as needed.
- Develop and implement explicit strategies for achieving consistent nutritional care by various providers.
- Communicate to other professionals and families the importance of nutrition and of special nutritional interventions in the promotion or improvement of health.

- Organize in-service education programs for care providers to address complex nutritional problems during and after pregnancy.
- Plan and implement activities to evaluate the quality of nutritional care and the safety and effectiveness of the nutrition program.

SUMMARY

Basic nutrition services can and should be integrated into the routine health care of expectant and new mothers by physicians, midwives, nurses, and dietitians. Experts should be involved in providing prenatal and postnatal services to women with health problems that require complex diet modification or nutritional support. This ordinarily requires a coordinated effort by an experienced multidisciplinary team composed of a physician, a nurse, a dietitian, and perhaps several other specialists.

REFERENCES

1. Food and Nutrition Service, U.S. Department of Agriculture. 1985. Part 246.2–Special Supplemental Food Program For Women, Infants and Children: definitions. Federal Register 50(30):6121.
2. Chapman, J., E. Siegel, and A. Cross. 1990. Home visitors and child health: analysis of selected programs. Pediatrics 85:1059-1068.
3. National Commission to Prevent Infant Mortality. 1989. Home Visiting: Opening Doors for America's Pregnant Women and Children. National Commission to Prevent Infant Mortality, Washington, D.C.
4. Olds, D.L., and H. Kitzman. 1990. Can home visitation improve the health of women and children at environmental risk? Pediatrics 86:108-116.
5. General Accounting Office. 1990. Home Visiting: A Promising Early Intervention Strategy for At-Risk Families. GAO Publ. No. HRD-90-83. General Accounting Office, Washington, D.C.
6. Institute of Medicine. 1992. Nutrition During Pregnancy and Lactation: An Implementation Guide. Report of the Subcommittee for a Clinical Applications Guide, Committee on Nutritional Status During Pregnancy and Lactation. Food and Nutrition Board. National Academy Press, Washington, D.C.
7. Peoples-Sheps, M.D., W.D. Kalsbeek, E. Siegel, C. Dewees, M. Rogers, and R. Schwartz. 1991. Prenatal records: a national survey of content. Am. J. Obstet. Gynecol. 164:514-521.
8. Macro Systems, Inc. 1990. One-Stop Shopping for Perinatal Services: Identification and Assessment of Implementation Methodologies. National Center for Education in Maternal and Child Health, Washington, D.C.
9. Hill, I.T., and J. Breyel. 1989. Coordinating Prenatal Care. National Governors' Association, Washington, D.C.
10. Tindall, J.A. 1989. Peer Counseling: In-Depth Look At Training Peer Helpers, 3rd ed. Accelerated Development Inc., Muncie, Ind.

11. Institute of Medicine. 1990. Nutrition During Pregnancy: Weight Gain and Nutrient Supplements. Report of the Subcommittee on Nutritional Status and Weight Gain During Pregnancy and the Subcommittee on Dietary Intake and Nutrient Supplements During Pregnancy, Committee on Nutritional Status During Pregnancy and Lactation, Food and Nutrition Board. National Academy Press, Washington, D.C.
12. Boisvert-Walsh, C., and J. Kallio. 1990. Reaching out to those at highest risk. Pp. 63-84 in M. Kaufman, ed. Nutrition in Public Health. Aspen Publishers, Rockville, Md.

4

Basic Nutrition Services for Newborn Infants

BASIC CARE FOR THE NEONATE

Exclusive breastfeeding is the preferred method of feeding normal infants throughout their first 4 to 6 months. Breastfeeding provides the infant with a clean supply of milk, in an amount that is responsive to the infant's needs, and in a manner that promotes optimal interaction between the mother and infant. Human milk provides all essential nutrients in a form that is easily digested and absorbed and in amounts that allow normal growth and development of full-term infants (assuming adequate exposure to sunlight). Moreover, human milk provides the infant with immunoglobulins and many other antiinfective substances, as well as anti-inflammatory substances, hormones, enzymes, and growth factors that appear to have important health-promoting effects. It also appears to minimize the risk of allergic reactions. Breastfeeding may benefit the mother by suppressing ovulation (thereby extending the period of postpartum infertility), hastening the return of the uterus to its prepregnant size (which reduces the risk of hemorrhage in the immediate postpartum period), and perhaps reducing the risk of certain health problems (such as osteoporosis and breast cancer) later in life.[1]

The approach to basic nutritional care of the neonate presented in this chapter is consistent with national health goals for the year 2000:

> Increase to at least 75 percent the proportion of mothers who breastfeed their babies in the early postpartum period and to at least 50 percent the proportion who continue breastfeeding until their babies are 5 to 6 months old (p. 123).[2]

Breastfeeding rates in 1988 were very much lower than this at discharge from the birth site: 54% for white mothers, 32% for low-income mothers, 25% for black mothers, and 51% for Hispanic mothers.[2] Rates for migrant Hispanic mothers appear to be lower than those for nonmigrants.[3]

When breastfeeding is not desired or not possible, modern infant formulas are an acceptable alternative if they are prepared and fed properly. The committee strongly endorses breastfeeding. It also believes that each woman should be able to make an informed decision about which feeding method will be most acceptable for her situation and to receive nutrition services appropriate to that choice. For example, the woman who decides to feed her baby formula may need to be taught how to reconstitute it. The committee supports a patient-centered plan of care to promote appropriate infant feeding.

Planning for the Support of the Breastfeeding Woman

Nutritional care of the breastfed infant mainly involves breastfeeding support for the mother. Most women make decisions about how to feed their infant before or during pregnancy.[4,5] A small randomized study demonstrated that prenatal breastfeeding education was associated with higher rates of breastfeeding by low-income African-American women than by their counterparts in a control group.[6] Thus, information to support the decision to breastfeed should be provided preconceptionally and prenatally, and methods to convey the information need to consider outside influences on decision making.[7] Women may benefit from practical information about how to breastfeed offered during prenatal visits or classes as well as in the immediate postpartum period.

The logical times for health care providers to provide direct assistance to and support for the breastfeeding mother are when she first initiates feedings and when her milk "comes in." Advice and support are also needed for mothers who encounter difficulties or have concerns in the following weeks or months. Hospitals should implement standard practices that facilitate the initiation of breastfeeding (such as those described by Strembel and colleagues,[8] Winikoff and others,[9] and the World Health Organization)[10], and primary care providers need to offer additional services after discharge. (See also Spisak and Gross.[11])

During their hospitalization, women who deliver vaginally usually have only a short period to acquire breastfeeding skills and to ask questions. In 1990, the mean duration of hospitalization for these women, including time spent in labor, was 2.4 days (E. Graves, National Center for Health Statistics, personal communication, 1991); many women are discharged within 24 to 36 hours after delivery. Fatigue or discomfort during the hospital stay may temporarily interfere with the mother's learning. Mothers whose infants are delivered by cesarean section have longer hospital stays (mean = 4.6 days) and thus more opportunity for interactions. However, such women require extra assistance and support from skilled nursing staff to manage the discomforts and other barriers to breastfeeding that result from this major surgery, including the likelihood of greater separation from the newborn infant while in the hospital.[12-14]

Breastfeeding women who return to work or school are usually confronted with barriers to breastfeeding. Health care providers can assist them (1) by helping with practical details such as how to pump and store milk and (2) by providing information to the worksite about the advantages of supporting breastfeeding and about helpful short-term strategies, such as alterations in work schedules and a private place for expressing milk.[15,16] To make breastfeeding a more realistic option for women after they leave the hospital or birth center will require greater community acceptance of and tangible support for breastfeeding as the preferred method of feeding babies.

To provide women with adequate support for breastfeeding involves activities of many types:

- For both health care providers and the general population, raising the level of awareness of breastfeeding as an infant feeding option—this could be carried out as a part of both women's health and school-based health education.
- Education and training for health care personnel in policies, procedures, and skills that promote and support breastfeeding.
- Educational activities for parents (such as prenatal and early postpartum classes, demonstrations, and videotapes) about the benefits and techniques of breastfeeding.
- The discontinuation of hospital practices (such as distributing infant formula gift packages) that tend to undermine breastfeeding.
- Early and direct assistance with breastfeeding upon its initiation in the hospital and as needed during the hospital stay.
- Skilled nursing care to assist women with breastfeeding following a cesarean delivery.
- Instructions for contacting the physician in the event of breastfeeding or infant health problems and encouragement to do so. For example, early symptoms of mastitis, decisions concerning prescription medications for the mother, and concerns about the adequacy of the infant's intake should be directed to the physician as soon as possible.
- Specific information before discharge about sources of support for the process of breastfeeding. Such sources include La Leche League,

Mothers of Twins, other mother-to-mother support groups, a telephone hot line for breastfeeding women, or the hospital's lactation consultant.

- Support for and additional information about breastfeeding provided in the woman's home within a few days after discharge.
- Support for and additional information about breastfeeding at the first neonatal health visit (within 2 weeks after birth)[17] and at the routine postpartum visit, with anticipatory guidance to prevent premature cessation of breastfeeding.[18]
- Assistance with strategies for continuing to breastfeed upon returning to work or school.

Home Visits and Other Early Follow-up

The home visit deserves special consideration and discussion because it is not a part of routine care in the United States. In Western Europe, home visits (usually by specially trained nurses) are widely used in postnatal care: seven of nine countries always provided at least one postnatal home visit in 1982.[19] In the United States, the value of home visits for a variety of purposes is receiving increasing recognition.[20-30]

Home visits offer unique opportunities for care providers to observe infant feeding and care practices, the mother's coping skills, and the resources available to the mother; they also allow follow-up of many other aspects of maternal and infant health. Such observations enable the home visitor to tailor the assistance and educational strategies to the mother's and infant's special needs. Suitably trained home visitors can quickly identify ways to advise the mother on planning simple but nutritious meals and snacks, avoiding or managing infant feeding problems, and resolving other concerns. This may be especially valuable for mothers of twins, low-income women, adolescents, women with limited education or intelligence, and women with a history of problems with child rearing. The home visit is also an opportunity to provide direct assistance with techniques for the manual expression of milk and, if desired, for the use of a breast pump.

Although too few studies have been conducted to allow an adequate evaluation of the cost-effectiveness of postpartum home visits, the U.S. General Accounting Office concluded that "home visiting is a promising strategy for delivering or improving access to early intervention services that can help at-risk families become healthier and more self-sufficient" (p. 2).[29] A telephone contact can serve as only a partial substitute for a home visit because it does not allow for direct observation or intervention, or for the modeling of desirable behaviors.

A home or office visit with a physician, midwife, or nurse-practitioner within approximately 2 weeks of delivery is highly desirable for both medical follow-up of the neonate and the support of either breastfeeding or appropriate formula feeding. Early discharge (<48 hours after delivery) calls for earlier follow-up.[17]

DELIVERY OF BASIC NUTRITION SERVICES FOR INFANTS

Availability of the following nutrition services is basic to the preparation of parents for infant care, to the care of all normal infants, and to the care of previously ill or disabled infants who have been discharged to routine care. (See also Chapter 3 for information about services in support of breastfeeding.)

- Offer or organize structured programs to provide information about infant feeding choices to pregnant women and their partners and to support breastfeeding efforts in the hospital and following discharge.
- Provide support for and assistance to breastfeeding mothers as described in the preceding section "Planning for the Support of the Breastfeeding Woman." This may include special support for mothers of twins or triplets and for those who plan to continue breastfeeding after returning to work or school.
- Evaluate and manage the nutritional care of the infant.
  - Screen for nutrition-related problems such as phenylketonuria, over- or underfeeding, inappropriate feedings or nutrient supplements, and abnormal patterns of growth.
  - Measure, monitor, and assess infant growth.
  - Provide instructions for the safe preparation of infant formula, feeding instructions, and anticipatory guidance for the primary caregiver and others as appropriate.
  - Address feeding practices to prevent the development of tooth decay in infants.
  - Determine the need to adjust feeding strategies, formula (if used), and vitamin-mineral supplements.
  - Adjust recommendations to treat food- and nutrition-related problems of the infant, such as overnutrition, undernutrition, anemia, and allergies.
  - Consult with specialists concerning complex nutritional challenges (see Chapter 5) and make referrals as necessary.
- Provide for the continuity of nutritional care; this includes referral to and communications with outpatient and home health services and parental support groups, as well as referral to local agencies with food and nutrition programs (see Chart 3-2) when appropriate.

- Provide organized in-service nutrition education for the health care team about normal nutrition throughout the first years of life.

Personnel

The health care team may include physicians (pediatricians or family practitioners with special interest in the care of the newborn), midwives, nurse-practitioners, nurses (hospital based or in the physician's office), and sometimes a dietitian or a social worker, or both. These team members need experience in providing for the nutritional needs of lactating mothers (see Chapter 3) and in the feeding of newborn infants. They also need to be familiar with sources of assistance in the community, their eligibility requirements, and strategies for helping parents gain access to these sources. It is essential that all members of the team convey consistent, accurate messages to the mother about infant growth, nutrition, and feeding techniques.

Nurses are expected to be able to provide support and technical assistance in the art of breastfeeding and to help find solutions to common problems that might otherwise obstruct successful breastfeeding. The nurse, nurse-practitioner, midwife, and physician are the caregivers who are primarily responsible for teaching the mother about the care of her infant.

Ancillary personnel in the community extend the reach and effectiveness of the facility-based health care team. For example, if the Expanded Food and Nutrition Education Program (EFNEP) is available locally, a nutrition teaching aide can help low-income families stretch their food dollars and make more healthful food choices during lactation; a visiting nurse can provide breastfeeding support and assist the mother in the safe handling of her expressed milk or of formula; and a community health worker may help link the mother with needed resources. WIC staff can offer helpful information on food choices during lactation and on breastfeeding management for those women who are enrolled in the program.

Knowledge Base and Clinical Skills

Health care providers who are responsbile for the nutritional care of normal infants and of breastfeeding mothers are expected to have a firm knowledge base concerning the following topics and the education and experience needed to develop the skills covered in this section.

Knowledge and Understanding

- Similarities and differences in the composition of human milk and infant formulas.
- Factors that facilitate or hinder successful breastfeeding.
- Methods for overcoming barriers to breastfeeding, both at home and after the mother returns to work or school.
- Practical information about breastfeeding techniques, such as positioning the baby.
- Conditions that require the physician's attention, including early signs of mastitis, dehydration of the infant, abnormally slow infant growth, or unadvised discontinuation of a prescription medicine.
- Nutrient requirements of normal infants at each stage of development and appropriate ways to provide those nutrients.
- Neuromuscular development related to the appropriate times for the introduction of solid foods and the emergence of self-feeding.
- Safety precautions for formula preparation.

Assessment Skills

- Obtain a current feeding history.
- Identify barriers to the continuation of breastfeeding.
- Identify the mother's strengths and the resources available to her—to serve as a basis for a constructive plan of care.
- Accurately measure the infant and monitor his or her weight and length.
- Detect abnormal growth and developmental patterns.
- Determine the need for adjustments in the feeding program.
- Identify the need for referral for special nutritional care for the infant.

Health Maintenance Skills

- Provide nutrition education and counseling that is appropriate for the feeding method chosen. This may include information regarding the management of successful breastfeeding, hygienic measures for the safe handling and feeding of formula and supplementary foods, the appropriate use of infant formula, the indications for and safe use of nutrient supplements, the supplementation of breastfeeding or formula with other foods or fluids, the prevention of baby bottle-mouth syndrome, or any combination of these.

- Provide support and technical assistance in the art of breastfeeding and in coping with other aspects of infant feeding.
- Communicate in a second language or make effective use of an interpreter or translator to communicate with non-English-speaking families.

Intervention Skills

- Use problem-solving techniques to support breastfeeding women who may otherwise wean their babies prematurely.
- Manage the nutritional care of infants with health problems who have been discharged to routine care.
- Assist the caregiver to solve real or perceived feeding problems.
- Facilitate the parents' use of available community services and agencies that provide resources to support maternal and child nutrition.

Management of the Organization and Delivery of Nutritional Care

- Assist in training home visitors (including peer counselors) to support breastfeeding and to provide guidance on other aspects of infant feeding.
- Develop strategies for achieving consistency of care by various health team members and for triggering appropriate follow-up when there is a change in providers.
- Incorporate new knowledge into nutritional care plans and educational programs.

SUMMARY

Because exclusive breastfeeding is the recommended feeding method for infants for the first 4 to 6 months, basic nutritional care for the neonate needs increased attention to support for breastfeeding, preferably beginning before conception. Emphasis should be placed on appropriate anticipatory guidance both pre- and postnatally, direct support in the hospital, and a variety of forms of assistance with breastfeeding management after discharge. Early home visits offer a promising strategy for supporting continued breastfeeding.

REFERENCES

1. Institute of Medicine. 1991. Nutrition During Lactation. Report of the Subcommittee on Nutrition During Lactation, Committee on Nutritional Status During Pregnancy and Lactation, Food and Nutrition Board. National Academy Press, Washington, D.C.
2. Department of Health and Human Services. 1990. Healthy People 2000: National Health Promotion and Disease Prevention Objectives. Public Health Service, Office of the Assistant Secretary for Health, Washington, D.C.
3. O'Malley, B., A.C. Brown, M. Tate, A.A. Hertzler, and M.H. Rojas. 1991. Infant feeding practices of migrant farm laborers in northern Colorado. J. Am. Diet. Assoc. 91:1084-1087.
4. Hally, M.R., J. Bond, J. Crawley, B. Gregson, P. Philips, and I. Russell. 1984. Factors influencing the feeding of first-born infants. Acta. Paediatr. Scand. 73:33-39.
5. Sarett, H.P., K.R. Bain, and J.C. O'Leary. 1983. Decisions on breast-feeding or formula feeding and trends in infant-feeding practices. Am. J. Dis. Child 137:719-725.
6. Kistin, N., D. Benton, S. Rao, and M. Sullivan. 1990. Breastfeeding rates among black urban low-income women: effect of prenatal education. Pediatrics 86:741-746.
7. Baranowski, T., D.E. Bee, D.K. Rassin, C.J. Richardson, J.P. Brown, N. Guenther, and P.R. Nader. 1983. Social support, social influence, ethnicity and the breastfeeding decision. Soc. Sci. Med. 17:1599-1611.
8. Strembel, S., S. Sass, G. Cole, and J. Hartner. 1991. Breast-feeding policies and routines among Arizona hospitals and nursery staff: results and implications of a descriptive study. J. Am. Diet. Assoc. 91:923-925.
9. Winikoff, B., D. Myers, V.H. Laukaran, and R. Stone. 1987. Overcoming obstacles to breast-feeding in a large municipal hospital: applications of lessons learned. Pediatrics 80:423-433.
10. World Health Organization. 1989. Protecting, Promoting and Supporting Breast-feeding: The Special Role of Maternity Services. A Joint WHO/UNICEF Statement. World Health Organization, Geneva.
11. Spisak, S., and S.S. Gross. 1991. Second Followup Report: The Surgeon General's Workshop on Breastfeeding and Human Lactation. National Center for Education in Maternal and Child Health, Washington, D.C.
12. Frantz, K.B., and B.A. Kalmen. 1979. Breastfeeding works for cesareans, too. RN 42(12):39-47.
13. Lawrence, R.A. 1989. Breastfeeding: A Guide for the Medical Profession, 3rd ed. C.V. Mosby, St. Louis.
14. Nurses Association of the American College of Obstetricians and Gynecologists. 1991. Facilitating Breastfeeding. NAACOG, Washington, D.C.
15. Barber-Madden, R., M.A. Petschek, and J. Pakter. 1987. Breastfeeding and the working mother: barriers and intervention strategies. J. Public Health Pol. 8:531-541.
16. Petschek, M.A., and R. Barber-Madden. 1985. Promoting prenatal care and breastfeeding in the workplace. Occ. Health Nurs. 33:86-89.
17. American Academy of Pediatrics/American College of Obstetricians and Gynecologists. 1992. Guidelines for Perinatal Care, 3rd ed. American Academy of Pediatrics, Elk Grove, Ill.
18. Ferris, A.M., L.T. McCabe, L.H. Allen, and G.H. Pelto. 1987. Biological and sociocultural determinants of successful lactation among women in eastern Connecticut. J. Am. Diet. Assoc. 87:316-321.
19. Miller, C.A. 1988. Prenatal care outreach: an international perspective. Pp. 210-228 in S. Brown, ed. Prenatal Care: Reaching Mothers, Reaching Infants. National Academy Press, Washington, D.C.
20. Aaronson, M. 1989. The case manager-home visitor. Child Welfare 68:339-346.

21. Chapman, J., E. Siegel, and A. Cross. 1990. Home visitors and child health: analysis of selected programs. Pediatrics 85:1059-1068.
22. Combs-Orme, T., J. Reis, and L.D. Ward. 1985. Effectiveness of home visits by public health nurses in maternal and child health: an empirical review. Public Health Rep. 100:490-499.
23. Heins, H.C., N.W. Nance, and J.E. Ferguson. 1987. Social support in improving perinatal outcome: the Resource Mothers Program. Obstet. Gynecol. 70:263-266.
24. Klerman, L.V. 1990. Home visiting during pregnancy. Pp. 593-602 in I.R. Merkatz and J.E. Thompson, eds. New Perspectives on Prenatal Care. Elsevier, New York.
25. Larson, C.P. 1980. Efficacy of prenatal and postpartum home visits on child health and development. Pediatrics 66:191-197.
26. National Commission to Prevent Infant Mortality. 1989. Home Visiting: Opening Doors for America's Pregnant Women and Children. National Commission to Prevent Infant Mortality, Washington, D.C.
27. Olds, D., C. Henderson, R. Tatelbaum, and R. Chamberlin. 1986. Improving the delivery of prenatal care and outcomes of pregnancy: a randomized trial of nurse home visitation. Pediatrics 77:16-28.
28. Olds, D.L., and H. Kitzman. 1990. Can home visitation improve the health of women and children at environmental risk? Pediatrics 86:108-116.
29. Powell, D.R. 1990. Home visiting in the early years: policy and program design decisions. Young Children 45:65-73.
30. General Accounting Office. 1990. Home Visiting: A Promising Early Intervention Strategy for At-Risk Families. GAO Publ. No. HRD-90-83. General Accounting Office, Washington, D.C.

5

Newborns Who Need Special Nutritional Care

Adequate nutrition is a cornerstone of the care of newborns and older infants with serious health problems or disabilities. Such infants present many challenges to the health team members responsible for their nutritional care. They may have difficulties with feeding per se, or they may have physiologic problems that call for specialized nutrition support to achieve their nutritional goals, including appropriate growth and development, while avoiding potential complications associated with feeding. This chapter has four objectives: (1) to provide information about high-risk neonates and the challenges they present, (2) to describe briefly the variety of feeding methods used for these infants, (3) to summarize the complex monitoring required, and (4) to discuss nutrition service delivery for this population.

BACKGROUND

Conditions That Often Require Special Nutritional Care

Many newborn infants require hospitalization for extended periods because of problems associated with preterm birth (gestational age at birth, ≤37 weeks), low birth weight (LBW; <2,500 g), or very low birth weight (VLBW; <1,500 g). The rates of LBW and VLBW among infants born in

CHART 5-1 Examples of Conditions That Require Special Nutrition Management of the Neonate

- Prematurity (≤37 weeks' gestational age)[a]
- Very low birth weight (less than 1,500 g)[a]
- Low birth weight (less than 2,500 g)[a]
- Congenital anomalies of the gastrointestinal, renal, hepatic, cardiovascular, and central nervous systems
- Oral-facial anomalies, e.g., cleft palate
- Some congenital syndromes and genetic disorders, e.g., cystic fibrosis and Down syndrome
- Inborn errors of metabolism, e.g., phenylketonuria (PKU), galactosemia, or maple sugar urine disease (MSUD)
- Necrotizing enterocolitis
- Excessive or intractable diarrhea or vomiting
- Respiratory distress or apnea
- Chronic lung disease (bronchopulmonary dysplasia)
- Maternal diabetes mellitus
- Drug withdrawal
- Sepsis, peritonitis, meningitis
- Perinatal hypoxia

[a]The complexity of the nutritional concerns increases with decreasing length of gestation and birth weight.

the United States are high compared with the rates in other industrialized countries. These rates are especially high among disadvantaged groups; for example, LBW and VLBW rates for African-Americans were 12.7% and 2.7%, respectively, in 1987.[1] The use of illegal drugs, especially cocaine, contributes to the problem of low birth weight[2] and is associated with decreased head circumference.[3]

Although a majority of the infants who require intensive care are born preterm or very small, others are full-term infants with serious congenital birth defects or with any of a large number of other conditions that require special nutritional management (see Chart 5-1). The wide range of problems and the differences among infants make it essential to set individualized nutrition goals for each child.

Challenges That Confront Clinicians

Establishing goals for compromised neonates is often a complex process.[4,5] Nutritional goals for these infants may be substantially different from those for healthy full-term infants because they must be adjusted for gestational age, postnatal age, medical condition, and route of feeding. Technical problems, such as intravenous access in small infants, inability to maintain nutrient solubility, and drug-nutrient interactions may further complicate nutritional support. It is inappropriate and sometimes hazardous simply to apply approaches used for adults to the care of neonates.[6]

Estimating Nutrient Requirements

Estimating the nutrient requirements of neonates with special needs is a challenge. Providing too little or too much of even a single nutrient may prevent or retard growth or result in serious physiologic problems. Recommended Dietary Allowances (RDAs)[7] are of limited usefulness for estimating the nutrient needs of neonates. (RDAs are defined as the levels of intake of essential nutrients that, on the basis of scientific knowledge, are judged by the Food and Nutrition Board to be adequate to meet the known nutrient needs of practically all *healthy* persons.) For young infants, the RDAs are based on a weight of 6 kg, with only one RDA per nutrient spanning the first 6 months after birth. Thus, they are not intended to describe the individual nutrient needs of healthy newborn infants, nor are they intended for infants who are stressed by illness or surgery, whose activity is affected by a disability, or who were born at early gestational ages. Infants with bronchopulmonary dysplasia, a chronic respiratory disease common in premature infants, illustrate one kind of change in requirements that may result from illness: such infants may expend as much as 25% more energy than normal infants.[8]

In part because published information on desirable intakes is incomplete, considerable judgment is required in deciding on appropriate amounts of certain nutrients for neonates—especially amounts of protein;[9] vitamins A,[10] D, and E; and calcium, phosphate,[11,12] and iron.[13] This uncertainty, in turn, increases the importance of frequent, individualized monitoring to determine whether adjustments in intake are needed. Such monitoring is essential to maintain an individualized, patient-centered care plan.

Adapting to Changing Needs

A second challenge relates to rapid changes in the infant's needs—only some of which are related to growth. For example, VLBW infants may experience wide variations in energy metabolism and may demonstrate rapid changes in their needs for water, solutes, or both.[14] Rapid changes in medical status may be accompanied by further changes in nutrient needs. These changes call for increased monitoring to determine the appropriateness of nutritional therapy.

Physical and Physiologic Limitations

A third challenge relates to the infant's physical limitations, especially in gastrointestinal function. Premature, sick, and handicapped infants may be unable to handle feedings by mouth or tube, or they may be able to tolerate only special infant formulas. Innovations in nutrient delivery, along with improved formulations, have been responsible for much progress in neonatal nutrition. For example, parenteral nutrition has been life saving for many infants who are unable to tolerate enteral feedings (see, e.g., Goulet and colleagues[15]). However, this feeding method is accompanied by increased risk of such conditions as hyperglycemia, hyperlipidemia, and life-threatening infections, and the possibility of mechanical catheter complications. Continuous tube feedings have helped many infants; however, tube feeding exposes the infant to other risks—for example, gastrointestinal perforation and aspiration. A further concern is either toxicity or metabolic complications, which may result from excessive or unbalanced intakes of such nutrients as water, protein, calcium, and trace elements (e.g., zinc), and possibly from aluminum.[16]

Effects of Medical Therapies on Nutrition

A fourth challenge is presented by the effects of medical therapies on the infant's nutrient needs and tolerance to feeding. The use of some drugs (e.g., diuretics) may cause mineral losses; dialysis affects the need for fluids and for certain other nutrients; hypertonic medications may lead to vomiting, diarrhea, and, in some cases, necrotizing enterocolitis; methods of delivering oxygen support may limit enteral feeding options; and infant warmers for LBW babies increase fluid requirements. Long-term parenteral nutrition has been associated with cholestasis.

Successful interventions require a well-trained, highly skilled team of personnel. They also necessitate close observation and frequent monitoring of both biochemical and anthropometric parameters and of feeding tolerance.

The Nutritional Care Plan

An individualized nutritional care plan is needed for each infant requiring specialized nutritional care. Participants in such planning should include the parent(s) and other persons they designate as key providers of support, as well as the traditional health care team. If there is a language barrier, a skilled interpreter is needed to help with communication. The care plan should address the infant's feedings (what is to be fed, how it is to be fed, and how often), the methods to be used to monitor the infant's progress, the kinds of education and other forms of support that the parents will need to participate actively in the nutritional care of their child, and referrals to appropriate caregivers and agencies. In addition, the plan should make certain that all routine newborn laboratory screening tests (e.g., for PKU) are performed and that the results are followed up.

Support for the parents may involve the use of community resources, such as early intervention programs, as well as inpatient and outpatient services. Home visits by nurses or other trained health care workers would help in tailoring the plan of care and the teaching strategies to the needs and resources of the family, as well as to the specific home environment.

Parents of preterm or developmentally delayed infants need assistance to develop realistic expectations for the infant's growth and development.[17] For example, adjustments are made for the young gestational age of preterm infants when anticipating developmental milestones that relate to feeding (such as the development of coordinated tongue movements or of sucking and swallowing).

FEEDING METHODS

There are two general approaches to the feeding of small, sick, or handicapped newborn infants: enteral feeding and parenteral feeding. Enteral feeding makes use of the gastrointestinal tract; it may involve feeding by mouth or by feeding tube. Parenteral feeding involves supplying nutrients through peripherally or centrally placed intravenous catheters. Parenteral feeding is undertaken only when it is impossible to provide adequate nutrition enterally. In many cases, infants are supported initially with parenteral feedings and then are adapted gradually to enteral feedings.

Each enteral and parenteral method has specific indications, contraindications, requirements, and complications.[18-20] This section describes these methods and feedings briefly, indicates key decisions, and illustrates the complexity of nutritional management of high-risk neonates.

Enteral Feedings

Human Milk

For many infants who require specialized nutritional care, human milk is preferred as the major source of nutrients. Depending on the condition of the infant, human milk may be fed by breastfeeding, bottle, tube, or a combination of these methods. Although milk from the mothers of preterm infants tends to be higher in protein than milk obtained from mothers of full-term infants, it does not provide sufficient quantities of protein or of other nutrients to meet the increased requirements of growing VLBW infants, of infants who are small for gestational age, and of infants experiencing certain other kinds of stress. In such cases, expressed mother's milk or milk from a human milk bank[a] can be fortified with commercial human milk fortifiers or other sources of nutrients.[21-23] Fortified mother's milk provides the infant with a wide array of protective substances that are not present in formula.[24,25] Lucas and Cole[26] present evidence from a large, randomized trial that feeding human milk may help prevent necrotizing enterocolitis.

Mothers who are taking certain drugs, who are critically ill themselves, or who have certain infectious diseases may be unable to provide adequate or safe milk. For example, the Centers for Disease Control[27] and *Guidelines for Perinatal Care*[28] have advised against breastfeeding by U.S. mothers who test positive for the human immunodeficiency virus (HIV). More commonly, practical barriers (such as long travel times between home and the neonatal intensive care unit and the difficulty of maintaining a milk supply without being able to nurse the baby) make it unrealistic for the mother to provide her milk for the infant.

If the mother chooses to provide her milk, she will need assistance in learning to pump her breasts or to express her milk manually; she will also need a private place to do so in the hospital (and at the worksite, if applicable) and information about how to store the milk properly to prevent contamination and the breakdown of nutrients. For short-term storage (≤48 hours), expressed human milk should be refrigerated; for longer storage, it should be frozen immediately. The mother who visits the hospital infrequently may send her frozen milk to the hospital between visits.

In the United States and Canada, there are few milk banks (eight in 1991). Milk from these banks differs in composition from that produced by individual mothers of premature infants, but it has been a satisfactory

---

[a]An organized unit that pools, pasteurizes, stores, and distributes human milk.

source of human milk if the milk has been fortified appropriately. Human milk banking is highly regulated because of concerns about HIV and other viruses. Pasteurization of human milk eliminates HIV and other viruses while moderately reducing the milk's health-promoting properties. The publication *Guidelines for the Establishment and Operation of a Human Milk Bank*[29] provides further information.

Formulas

If the feeding of human milk is not possible or desired, careful attention must be given to the selection of a formula that is appropriate for the newborn's gestational age and health status. Several formulas have been developed to meet the special nutritional needs of growing preterm infants.[30]

Specialty formulas address specific concerns, including lactose intolerance, increased vitamin and mineral requirements, impaired fat absorption, protein intolerance, and milk allergy. In fact, the choice of a formula for an individual infant with a specific set of needs becomes a technical decision. In view of the complexity of matching needs with formulas, a neonatal intensive care unit should have access to many formulas and additives, and an experienced team should be available to choose or design the optimal formula and vitamin-mineral supplementation regimen and to oversee the management of nutritional care.

In rare cases, an apparently healthy infant may have an inborn error of metabolism, such as PKU, that requires the feeding of a formula designed especially for treating the disorder. Treatment involves extended periods of special nutritional management, including close monitoring of the infant's serum phenylalanine values. This management is usually coordinated on an outpatient basis by a regional metabolic center. Parents may need assistance to obtain an adequate supply of the expensive formula.

Methods of Enteral Feeding

Breastfeeding

Premature or sick infants may be completely unable to breastfeed during the first days and weeks after birth. Convalescent infants and infants with handicaps may breastfeed more slowly or less efficiently and tire more easily than healthy full-term infants. Initially, many sick and premature infants may require total or supplemental feedings by gavage or intravenous routes to achieve adequate nutrient intake before breastfeeding can be fully established. Therefore, if the mother wants to be able to breastfeed fully when the infant is ready, she must learn to use a breast pump and receive guidance about its regular use; she must also learn to store her milk properly. In addition, she will need timely assistance in mastering techniques that facilitate adequate intake by infants with physical difficulties that complicate feeding,[31,32] and in achieving a pleasant, relaxed environment for expressing milk or for nursing.

Bottle Feeding

Bottle feeding of premature, sick, and handicapped infants is also more difficult than that of healthy full-term infants. When these infants are able to begin feedings, many have problems with the coordination of sucking, breathing, and swallowing. Careful assessment and intervention by the clinical team may be needed to assist with the oral feeding of both breastfed and bottlefed infants with oralfacial anomalies, those in whom the initiation of oral feeding is delayed for weeks, and postsurgical infants.

Scrupulous attention to detail is necessary in the preparation, storage, and handling of infant formulas of any type. These procedures are outlined in the book *Preparation of Formula for Infants: Guidelines for Health Care Facilities*.[33]

Tube Feeding

Inability to feed adequately either from breast or bottle is likely to be a problem for infants younger than 34 weeks of gestational age. The risk of aspiration may contraindicate oral feeding for infants of any age who have respiratory distress, abdominal distention, or tracheal-esophageal fistula. If the infant's gastrointestinal tract is functioning adequately, one of the following enteral feeding methods may be selected to provide his or her total nutrient intake or to supplement the infant's oral intake.

- Intermittent gavage feedings, in which a feeding catheter is passed either orally or nasally into the stomach.
- Continuous nasogastric feedings, which allow the infant to have a continuous infusion of milk or formula into the stomach.
- Gastrostomy feedings, in which a small opening is made surgically through the abdominal wall into the stomach to allow the direct insertion

of a feeding tube. Gastrostomy feedings may also be intermittent or continuous, depending on the infant's condition.

- Transpyloric feeding, in which feedings are provided through an indwelling catheter whose tip has passed through the stomach and pylorus into the small bowel (duodenum or jejunum). A transpyloric tube may be placed through a gastrostomy as needed.

The effects of different tube feeding methods are still under investigation (see, e.g., Grant and Denne[34]).

Gradual introduction of breastfeeding or bottle feeding for tube-fed infants is encouraged when the infant shows signs of readiness to suckle. At this time, the mother and infant will benefit from additional support in learning the art of feeding the infant with special needs. Supplemental tube feeding will continue until adequate oral intake can be achieved.

When the infant is unable to take any nourishment by nursing, it may be advisable to provide oral stimulation through the use of a pacifier or nipple to encourage sucking and the development of oral motor skills.

Parenteral Feeding

If the gastrointestinal tract cannot be used for feeding or can be used only to a limited extent, parenteral feeding assumes major importance. Although practices vary in different nurseries, many infants are not fed enterally while they are critically ill and so must rely on parenteral nutrition for all nutrients. However, nutritionally insignificant amounts of enteral feedings are sometimes given to stimulate intestinal function and growth and to reduce the likelihood of cholestasis.[35,36]

The intravenous infusion of amino acids, glucose, vitamins, minerals, trace elements, and fat emulsions requires careful control of the total volume and amounts of nutrients delivered (see, e.g., Greene et al.,[37] Hanning and Zlotkin,[38] and Heird et al.[39]). At any point in time, complex decisions concerning the appropriate formulation for an infant require the concerted, coordinated efforts of the neonatal team, which comprises the neonatologist, neonatal nurses and nurse-practitioners, a neonatal dietitian, and a pharmacist.[40] Information collected through careful monitoring (see the next section) is crucial to the decision-making process. Some infants—including those with congenital gastrointestinal anomalies, major gastrointestinal surgery, or complications related to necrotizing enterocolitis—may require prolonged parenteral nutrition (i.e., longer than 1 month). These infants are sometimes discharged on home parenteral nutrition if their families can successfully manage this complex feeding method.[41] Extensive training of parents is required, however, and these families need continuing support by a team experienced in the management of home parenteral nutrition for infants. It is important to recognize that not all families succeed in learning this technique.

With growth and maturation of the infant's gastrointestinal tract or improvement in the infant's medical condition, he or she may be weaned gradually from parenteral feedings while enteral feedings are being introduced and advanced.

MONITORING

Although all newborns should be monitored for the adequacy of nutritional intake, it is especially critical to monitor high-risk neonates frequently and with close attention to detail.[42-44] Such monitoring is described briefly below and is summarized in Chart 5-2.

Food and Fluid Intake and Output

An organized system for summarizing and tracking pertinent nutritional data is essential for adequate monitoring, efficient decision making, and other aspects of nutritional support. This system must be linked with detailed information about the composition of the infant's enteral and parenteral intake. Stave and colleagues[45] report on the value of such a system.

Most nurseries use a paper flow sheet to provide the required information in an easily accessible form. More recently, computerized systems, such as the one described by Lowe and colleagues,[46] are being used to organize data and generate progress notes. Collected data should include the daily volumes (intake) and the protein and energy values of enteral and parenteral fluids. The total fluid intake should be presented in relation to other data, such as the kinds and concentrations of formulas and supplements, the route of feeding of each, the amount fed, any gastric residuals, emesis, urine output, and stool frequency and description. To facilitate review, the data are presented in relation to the infant's weight.

Especially close monitoring of nutrient intake is needed when fluid intake must be restricted. Conditions requiring total fluid restriction include congestive heart failure, renal insufficiency, and chronic lung disease (bronchopulmonary dysplasia); limited gastric capacity requires restriction of enteral fluids.

CHART 5-2 Nutrition-Related Variables That May Need to Be Monitored for Newborns Who Require Special Care[a]

Nutrient intake
- Energy
- Protein
- Fluid

Growth variables
- Weight
- Length
- Head circumference

Metabolic variables
- Blood measurements
  - Plasma electrolytes
  - Plasma glucose
  - Triglycerides
  - Blood urea nitrogen
  - Plasma calcium, magnesium, phosphorus
  - Acid-base status
  - Serum protein (quantitative serum protein electrophoresis or albumin)
  - Liver function studies
  - Hemoglobin
- Urine glucose

Prevention and detection of infection
- Clinical observations (e.g., activity, temperature, abdominal tonicity)
- White blood cell count and differential
- Cultures

[a]The extent of monitoring and the frequency with which specific variables are monitored depend on the infant's gestational age, weight, medical condition, and feeding method.

For convalescent neonates, the observation of appropriate oral formula intake and adequate rates of gain in weight, length, and head circumference for gestational age provide good evidence of adequate nutrient intake.

Anthropometric Changes

The close monitoring of anthropometric changes is integral to the nutritional care of newborns. The postnatal growth patterns of newborns differ by both size and gestational age. Thus, an early step in monitoring anthropometric changes involves classifying the newborn infant.

Size categories for birth weight are adequate birth weight (≥2,500 g), LBW (<2,500 g), and, within the LBW group, VLBW (<1,500 g). Gestational age categories include preterm (≤37 weeks), full term (38 to 42 weeks), and post term (>42 weeks). Clinical obstetric estimation of gestational duration is based on maternal dates and on ultrasound examination. Gestational duration can also be estimated from physical examination of the infant, using the examinations by Dubowitz and colleagues[47] or Ballard and coworkers[48] for larger infants of more than 30 weeks' gestational age,[49] or using the more recent Ballard examination[50] for extremely low-birth-weight infants.

Reference values are available for normal birth weight, length, and head circumference at different gestational ages (see, e.g., Babson[51] and the review of growth curves by Sparks[5]). Based on the reference values used, infants are generally classified as appropriate for gestational age (AGA), small for gestational age (SGA), or large for gestational age (LGA).

Accurate anthropometric measurements made at appropriate intervals provide information that is crucial for clinical decision making in the intensive care unit (see, e.g., Kaempf and colleagues[52]). These measurements require that well-trained personnel use standardized techniques and accurate equipment, such as a well-calibrated digital scale. Quality control procedures should be in place to ensure accurate measurements over time.

It is important to plot changes in weight, length, and head circumference on appropriate grids. Adaptations of the classic weight curves by Dancis[53] are widely used for this purpose (see, e.g., Hay[4]). Other postnatal growth charts are available (e.g., Babson and Benda[54] and Gairdner and Pearson[55]). Alternatively, many centers plot longitudinal changes in length and head circumference on intrauterine charts (e.g., Lubchenco and colleagues[56]). Plotting the data facilitates the identification of infants who are growing slower or faster than the expected patterns. As with other nutrition-related decisions, such determinations may require sophisticated judgments by an experienced team.

Weight

Changes in weight over time provide a practical, relatively sensitive indicator of nutritional status, especially for LBW infants.[57] Nude weight should be recorded daily at a specific time, related to the feeding schedule, and plotted; this facilitates the identification of problems that require further evaluation and possible intervention. Full-term and SGA infants lose about 4% of their body weight after birth, with the maximum loss at 2 to 3 days. However, preterm infants may lose as much as 10 to 15% of their body weight by the end of the first week after birth, primarily because of extracellular fluid contraction.[58] Regular weighing of infants should be continued after discharge, with frequency depending on the extent of nutritional intervention and concern.

Length

The accurate and periodic measurement and plotting of length provides invaluable information about the infant's growth. For high-risk infants, it is important to measure length weekly in the hospital; however, for critically ill, intubated newborns, measurement of length may need to be delayed because of the risks involved in obtaining accurate measurements. Because the increase in length may be small relative to usual measurement errors, it is often difficult to assess change over short periods.

Head Circumference

Head circumference must also be measured, recorded, and plotted regularly, consistently, and accurately. As with length, increases in head circumference are small relative to potential measurement errors. If abnormal head growth is suspected, measurements should be made every 1 to 3 days in the hospital. Abnormalities include too little growth, raising concern about development of the brain, and too rapid growth, which may be indicative of hydrocephalus or intracranial hemorrhage. For VLBW infants, molding of the head may confuse the assessment of head growth.

At birth, the LBW infant's head may be small. Rapid increase in head circumference by 3 months of age may represent either desirable catch-up growth of the brain or excessive head growth resulting from hydrocephalus. It may be necessary to examine the infant's head with ultrasound, a computerized axial tomography (CAT) scan, or other techniques to determine the cause of rapid head growth.

Laboratory Values

The extent of monitoring of laboratory values depends on the infant's health status and feeding regimen. Preterm VLBW infants may benefit from routine laboratory monitoring of electrolytes, calcium, phosphorus, alkaline phosphatase, and hemoglobin and hematocrit. Additional variables may need to be monitored for special circumstances, such as parenteral feedings. Chart 5-3 lists many of the disorders that may result if feedings are not sufficiently individualized and adjusted to the infant's changing needs.

Clinical Observations

Careful, regular clinical observations—as of skin turgor, activity, and sleeping patterns—provide information that is important to the nutrition-related care of the newborn. Such observations are used, for example, in interpreting plots of weight change, because fluid retention or dehydration may have caused the change. Very subtle changes in the clinical appearance of a neonate may indicate serious and potentially fatal complications (such as sepsis), and they may signal a need to change the treatment plan, including method of feeding.

Monitoring of feeding tolerance is essential. This includes notation of the adequacy of the volume consumed, the occurrence of vomiting, the presence of residuals when the infant is tube fed, abdominal girth measurement, the frequency and character of the stools, and the presence or absence of a reducing substance in the stool.

NUTRITION SERVICES DELIVERY FOR NEONATES WITH SPECIAL NEEDS AND THEIR FAMILIES

Nutrition services for sick or recovering infants are delivered in diverse settings. In neonatal intensive care units and in intermediate care nurseries, skilled help is available. For convalescent infants, nutritional care is provided in other locations, such as the home, where trained personnel may be less available. This section describes the components of nutrition services required for these infants, the kinds of personnel needed to deliver them, and the knowledge base and skills required by personnel involved in the provision of intensive care, intermediate care, or convalescent care in the community.

CHART 5-3 Examples of Nutrition-Related Problems of Preterm Infants That Can Be Detected by Laboratory Tests

Iatrogenic disorders
- Hyperglycemia
- Hypoglycemia[a]
- Hyperlipidemia
- Azotemia[b]
- Electrolyte disorders
- Acid-base disorders
- Mineral (major and trace) disorders
- Vitamin disorders

Disorders caused by a suboptimal nitrogen source
- Acid-base disorder (hyperchloremic metabolic acidosis)
- Hyperammonemia
- Abnormal plasma aminograms

Hepatic disorders[c]
- Elevated transaminases
- Direct hyperbilirubinemia

Metabolic bone disease

[a]Often seen in infants of mothers with diabetes mellitus regardless of the feeding method.

[b]Also results from renal failure, regardless of the mode of feeding.

[c]Cholestasis is encountered frequently and is often accompanied by hyperbilirubinemia. The cause of this disorder is unknown, but it seems to be reversible in most cases.

Components of Special Nutrition Services

Intensive Care

Units that care for critically ill infants are responsible for providing a full range of appropriate resources and the expertise necessary to manage major newborn complications. A neonatal intensive care unit should be staffed and equipped to treat and provide nutritional support for critically ill infants and to facilitate the transition to a lower level of care, either in another hospital unit or at home. Many neonatal intensive care units are engaged in the teaching and training of medical students, interns, residents, nurses, and dietitians. They may also conduct research related to neonatal physiology, pathology, and nutrition. Detailed requirements for neonatal intensive care units are provided in *Guidelines for Perinatal Care*, published jointly by the American Academy of Pediatrics and the American College of Obstetricians and Gynecologists.[28]

Nutrition services for infants with special needs involve comprehensive nutritional care of the infant, facilitation of the family's participation in decision making and care, training and consultation for other care providers, and evaluation efforts. The elements of these services are summarized in the sections below.

Comprehensive Nutritional Care of the Neonate. Care of the neonate includes the initial nutritional assessment; screening for inborn errors of metabolism; developing and implementing comprehensive nutritional care plans (covering activities such as enteral and parenteral feedings, family involvement, and the monitoring of feeding tolerance, nutrient adequacy, and growth); and referrals as needed. Nutritional support should be assessed and the plan of care revised at least twice weekly while the infant is hospitalized and as needed after discharge.

Services for and Involvement of the Family. Optimal care of the newborn with special needs includes assisting family members to adjust to the situation and to learn the skills that will enable them to become active participants in the infant's care. Nursery staff can help the family to make such an adjustment and acquire the necessary skills by making the environment of the neonatal intensive care unit more inviting, and giving explanations, and initiating other measures that encourage parents to be with their infants. Among the many factors that contribute to an intimidating environment are a small, cramped space; high and distracting noise levels, especially if alarms sound frequently; and confusing visual stimuli, aggravated by complicated equipment. Good staff attitudes and improved facility design[59] may help to overcome these problems.

Families may need help to make informed decisions concerning enteral feeding of their newborn. They may also require assistance with techniques of breastfeeding, instructions for safe formula preparation and bottle feeding, demonstrations of oral stimulation, training on how to give tube or parenteral feedings, education and training to monitor the infant's progress, and education and counseling relating to realistic expectations and to the management of feeding problems.

Training and Consultation. Because of rapid changes in the field of infant nutrition, an organized in-service education program is invaluable for the health care team within the hospital and in the community. The neonatal health care team needs to be prepared to provide consultation services to facilities that provide less complex care and to train community personnel and family members to give follow-up care throughout the first year of life.

Evaluation. Ongoing evaluation of the nutrition program, including its safety and effectiveness, is essential to ensure high-quality care. At a programmatic level, the organized review of neonatal nutritional support services, with attention to usage, level of staff, and rate of nutrition-related complications, is an important part of quality assurance in a neonatal intensive care unit. Calculation of rates of nutrition-related complications provides an index for comparison with published estimates and may offer insight into the strengths and weaknesses of individual support services.

Intermediate Care

An intermediate care unit should be staffed and equipped to provide nutritional support for moderately ill infants or certain seriously ill infants who have been transferred out of intensive care because their conditions have stabilized. Often these infants need to feed and grow before discharge. Examples of conditions that require an intermediate level of care are mild respiratory distress syndrome, hyperbilirubinemia, hypoglycemia, medically stable VLBW, and mild infections. In addition, many infants with classical birth defects may be hospitalized in intermediate care units.

The services described previously for intensive care should be available in the intermediate care setting. However, because the infants being cared for in intermediate-level units have less complex conditions, the staff ordinarily handles routine decisions concerning nutritional management. In some situations, it is the intermediate care facility that has the major responsibility for teaching the family to assume full care of the infant upon discharge.

Follow-up Care in the Community

Infants with serious handicaps or other health problems may require specialized nutritional support (including monitoring) to achieve optimal growth and development even after discharge.[60] This applies to substantial numbers of premature infants: estimated rates of serious handicaps[b] for those surviving very low birth weights are 26% for those weighing <800 g at birth, 17% for those weighing 750 to 1,000 g, and 11% for those

[b]Serious handicaps are defined as one or more of the following: severe mental retardation (intelligence or development quotient below 70), cerebral palsy of significant degree, major seizure disorders, or blindness.

weighing 1,000 to 1,500 g.[61] A few seemingly normal infants may be found to have problems requiring specialized nutritional care after discharge. (See the previous subsection "Formulas.")

The follow-up care that is needed varies with the infant's condition, the family's capabilities, and the kinds of health services to which the family has access. Recommendations for follow-up should consider geographic location, as well as available transportation and other resources. Special early childhood intervention programs may help children who have serious health problems to reach their potential. In many communities, however, neither early intervention programs nor the services of specialized care providers are readily available. In this event, the care plan must match the needs of the infant and family with the available services and providers; it must also ensure that the providers receive appropriate guidance from specialists.

Personnel

The kinds of personnel necessary to provide neonatal nutrition services depend on the intensity of care required, but a multidisciplinary team is almost always essential. Appropriate staffing for nutrition services in intensive care nurseries includes neonatologists, who have the overall responsibility for the supervision, coordination, and delivery of primary neonatal care; neonatal nurses, who provide much of the direct care of the infant and family; a neonatal dietitian, who has a major role in the nutritional management of the infant; a clinical pharmacist, who deals with technical matters relating to feeding mixtures and supplements; a social worker, who provides much practical support for the family; an occupational therapist; a physical therapist; and a behavioral psychologist. A breastfeeding specialist and a speech and language pathologist (for oral motor evaluation and treatment) are also valuable resources.

In intermediate care centers, either the pediatrician or the neonatologist serves as the primary physician. This physician must be familiar with the nutritional limitations imposed by prematurity and birth defects, as well as the methods for dealing with the range of nutritional problems that are commonly encountered in the intermediate care nursery. For neonates with less serious disorders, pediatricians or neonatologists may serve as consultants to family physicians providing primary care to these newborns.

Regardless of the severity of the infant's condition, the neonatal nurse generally provides much of the direct care and often assumes the role of primary caregiver. The neonatal nurse is expected to develop great skill in using the many different feeding techniques; in monitoring the infant's intake, output, and feeding tolerance; and in interpreting the infant's progress in discussions with the parents.

The neonatal dietitian integrates information about the physiologic and biochemical bases for nutrient requirements (including changes by age, rate of growth, illness or surgery, and treatments) with information about the nutrient composition and other characteristics of feedings and feeding methods. The neonatal dietitian ordinarily coordinates, develops, implements, and evaluates an individualized plan for the provision of adequate inpatient nutritional care and facilitates the continuation of appropriate nutritional care following discharge. He or she may also participate in the education of other health care providers and students of the health professions.[62]

A pharmacist with expertise in the field of parenteral nutrition can make daily adjustments in the composition of parenteral feedings. He or she may also advise the other team members about special characteristics of parenteral feedings, the compatibility and stability of components of feedings, procedures for handling them, and drug-feeding interactions. Additional activities may be to check orders for accuracy and alert the team to new developments in parenteral feeding.

Education and Training of Health Care Providers

Because of the complexity of the nutritional problems that are encountered in neonatal intensive care and in many intermediate care nurseries, special training in neonatal nutrition is advisable for all health team members.

- The neonatologist should be a pediatrician who possesses active certification by the subspecialty board on neonatology of the American Board of Pediatrics. He or she should have experience with both short- and long-term implications and sequelae of the care of sick newborns. It is also desirable for the neonatologist to have participated in active clinical and research programs and to have an understanding of experimental design and methods of statistical evaluation of data. Recertification is a method to encourage updating of knowledge and skills.
- The nurse or nurse-practitioner should meet the qualifications necessary to function successfully in a newborn special care unit. However, he or she should also obtain additional in-service training in neonatal nutrition, feeding techniques and protocols, the system for collecting nutritional data, methods for monitoring nutritional progress, formula selection, and vitamin and mineral supplementation. Attendance at short courses in neonatal nutrition of 2 to 3 days' duration can increase the

nurse's appreciation of the need for careful nutrition monitoring and awareness of the nutrition-related roles of other team members in the neonatal unit.

- The neonatal dietitian should meet all the requirements for registration of the Council for Dietetic Registration and for licensure (where required); he or she should also have either advanced pediatric training that includes clinical neonatal nutrition or clinical experience in the nutritional care of critically ill newborn infants. Among the key areas for this training or experience are neonatal growth and development; nutritional assessment and monitoring; the influence of medical problems or treatment regimens on feeding; feeding alternatives, including neonatal parenteral nutrition; interactions among nutrients, drugs, and foods; the composition of feedings and supplements; and the education of family members and other care providers. Participation in a 3- to 6-month neonatal nutrition course is desirable for experienced dietitians to develop the special skills needed in the neonatal unit.
- It is desirable for the pharmacist to have completed an advanced degree or residency training in nutritional support pharmacy practice that meets the standards of the American Society of Hospital Pharmacists.[63] He or she should also obtain additional in-service training in relation to neonates.

Short refresher courses are a mechanism for updating knowledge and skills in this rapidly changing field.[62,64] Special conferences and courses in neonatal nutrition are valuable for educating clinicians about the scope and complexities of neonatal nutritional care and for developing skills in their respective areas. The science of human lactation and human milk should be included in these educational events.

Knowledge Base and Clinical Skills

For units that provide either intensive or intermediate neonatal care, the requisite knowledge base and clinical skills are generally similar. However, clinicians who work in an intermediate care unit can be somewhat less familiar with parenteral solutions and certain complex surgical and medical problems because they are likely to encounter less severe problems and only the more common kinds of medical and surgical conditions.

The team that provides nutrition services for infants with special nutritional needs and their families must have the knowledge and skills listed in Chapter 4 for basic nutrition services, plus those listed below.

Knowledge and Understanding

- Physiologic and biochemical bases of the nutrients required to support the growth of preterm and full-term infants.
- Relationships of infant development to infant feeding.
- Effects of complex medical and surgical problems on nutritional needs, on acceptable methods of feeding infants, and on potential complications of nutritional support regimens.
- Safe storage, handling, mixing, and delivery of human milk and infant formula.
- Appropriate nutritional therapies for disorders that affect the health or development of infants.
- Alternative feeding techniques for infants, the nutrient composition of specialized feedings (such as parenteral nutrition solutions and modified formulas), benefits and potential problems associated with the feeding methods, and principles involved in transitional feeding.

Assessment Skills

- Accurately measure length, weight, and head circumference.
- Identify abnormal patterns of growth and development of preterm and SGA infants and of infants with other health problems.
- Use appropriate screening, assessment, and monitoring methods to determine the nutritional progress of infants.
- Assess the family's capacity for participating in infant feeding and stimulation and for implementing a nutritional care plan after the infant's discharge.
- After discharge, obtain a nutrition history from the care providers that includes information about past and present feeding habits and responses, patterns of elimination, and the social setting associated with feeding.

Intervention Skills

- Manage and evaluate the nutritional care of seriously ill infants.
- Develop and participate in the implementation of appropriate nutritional care plans that consider the infant's developmental level; medical, surgical, or handicapping conditions; feeding techniques; and the nutrient content of feedings.
- Involve the family in the nutritional care of the infant during hospitalization.

• Provide nutrition counseling that enables parents or other primary caregivers to meet the nutritional needs of the patient.

• Function effectively as a multidisciplinary care team, recognizing that the services of many disciplines are essential for comprehensive care.

• Develop realistic nutritional care plans for meeting the infant's initial needs after discharge from the intensive or intermediate care nursery.

• Communicate to other professionals and parents the importance of nutrition to growth and health.

• Assist with case management, including plans for home visitation as needed.

Program Management and Evaluation Skills

• Provide organized nutrition education programs for the health care team in the hospital and in the community.

• Incorporate new knowledge into nutritional care plans, education programs, and protocols and procedures for the unit.

• Provide leadership in conducting activities to monitor and improve the quality and efficiency of the nutrition services being offered.

• Evaluate the results of nutrition-related interventions for use in program planning.

SUMMARY

Providing appropriate nutritional care for infants with special needs poses major challenges to clinicians and family members. A highly trained, multidisciplinary team is essential to provide the individualized care needed for satisfactory growth, development, and health of the infant when he or she requires intensive care. A team effort is also needed to help plan for appropriate follow-up care by primary care providers and family members during the infant's convalescence.

REFERENCES

1. National Center for Health Statistics. 1991. Health, United States, 1990. (PHS) 91-1232. U.S. Department of Health and Human Services, Hyattsville, Md.
2. Petitti, D.B., and C. Coleman. 1990. Cocaine and the risk of low birth weight. Am. J. Public Health 80:25-28.
3. Chasnoff, I.J., D.R. Griffith, C. Freier, and J. Murray. 1992. Cocaine/polydrug use in pregnancy: two-year follow-up. Pediatrics 89:284-289.

4. Hay, W.W. Jr., 1991. Nutritional needs of the extremely low-birth-weight infant. Semin. Perinatol. 15:482-492.
5. Sparks, J.W. 1984. Human intrauterine growth and nutrient accretion. Semin. Perinatol. 8:74-93.
6. Okken, A. 1991. Nutritional needs of newborn infants in intensive care. Int. J. Technol. Assess. Health Care 7(suppl. 1):94-98.
7. National Research Council. 1989. Recommended Dietary Allowances, 10th ed. Report of the Subcommittee on the Tenth Edition of the RDAs, Food and Nutrition Board, Commission on Life Sciences. National Academy Press, Washington, D.C.
8. Kurzner, S.I., M. Garg, D.B. Bautista, C.W. Sargent, C.M. Bowman, and T.G. Keens. 1988. Growth failure in bronchopulmonary dysplasia: elevated metabolic rates and pulmonary mechanics. J. Pediatr. 112:73-80.
9. Heird, W.C., S. Kashyap, and M.R. Gomez. 1991. Protein intake and energy requirements of the infant. Semin. Perinatol. 15:438-448.
10. Peeples, J.M., S.E. Carlson, S.H. Werkman, and R.J. Cooke. 1991. Vitamin A status of preterm infants during infancy. Am. J. Clin. Nutr. 53:1455-1459.
11. Hillman, L.S. 1990. Nutritional factors affecting mineral homeostasis and mineralization in the term and preterm infant. Pp. 55-92 in D.J. Simmons, ed. Nutrition and Bone Development. Oxford University Press, New York.
12. Koo, W.W., R.C. Tsang, P. Succop, S.K. Krug-Wispe, D. Babcock, and A.E. Oestreich. 1989. Minimal vitamin D and high calcium and phosphorus needs of preterm infants receiving parenteral nutrition. J. Pediatr. Gastroenterol. Nutr. 8:225-233.
13. Dallman, P.R. 1988. Nutritional anemia of infancy: iron, folic acid, and vitamin B_{12}. Pp. 216-235 in R.C. Tsang and B.L. Nichols, eds. Nutrition During Infancy. Hanley & Belfus, Philadelphia.
14. Baumgart, S. 1990. Water metabolism in the extremely-low-birth-weight infant. Pp. 83-93 in R.M. Cowett and W.W. Hay, Jr., eds. The Micropremie: The Next Frontier. Report of the Ninety-ninth Ross Conference on Pediatric Research. Ross Laboratories, Columbus, Ohio.
15. Goulet, O.J., Y. Revillon, D. Jan, S. De Potter, C. Maurage, S. Lortat-Jacob, H. Martelli, C. Nihoul-Fekete, and C. Ricour. 1991. Neonatal short bowel syndrome. J. Pediatr. 119:18-23.
16. Sedman, A.B., G.L. Klein, R.J. Merritt, N.L. Miller, K.O. Weber, W.L. Gill, H. Anand, and A.C. Alfrey. 1985. Evidence of aluminum loading in infants receiving intravenous therapy. N. Engl. J. Med. 312:1337-1343.
17. Field, T.M., S.M. Widmayer, S. Stringer, and E. Ignatoff. 1980. Teenage, lower-class, black mothers and their preterm infants: an intervention and developmental follow-up. Child Dev. 51:426-436.
18. Cowett, R.M., and W.W. Hay, Jr., eds. 1990. The Micropremie: The Next Frontier. Report of the Ninety-ninth Ross Conference on Pediatric Research. Ross Laboratories, Columbus, Ohio.
19. Hay, W.W., Jr., ed. 1991. Neonatal Nutrition and Metabolism. Mosby Year Book, St. Louis.
20. Klaus, M.H., and A.A. Fanaroff. 1986. Care of the High Risk Neonate, 3rd ed. W.B. Saunders Co., Philadelphia.
21. Greer, F.R., and A. McCormick. 1988. Improved bone mineralization and growth in premature infants fed fortified own mother's milk. J. Pediatr. 112:961-969.
22. Polberger, S.K.T., G.A. Fex, I.E. Axelsson, and N.C. Raiha. 1990. Eleven plasma proteins as indicators of protein nutritional status in very low birth weight infants. Pediatrics 86:916-921.
23. Schanler, R.J., and C. Garza. 1988. Improved mineral balance in very low birth weight infants fed fortified human milk. J. Pediatr. 112:452-456.

24. Institute of Medicine. 1991. Nutrition During Lactation. Report of the Subcommittee on Nutrition During Lactation, Committee on Nutritional Status During Pregnancy and Lactation, Food and Nutrition Board. National Academy Press, Washington, D.C.
25. Schanler, R.J. 1989. Human milk for preterm infants: nutritional and immune factors. Semin. Perinatol. 13:69-77.
26. Lucas, A., and T.J. Cole. 1990. Breast milk and neonatal necrotising enterocolitis. Lancet 336:1519-1523.
27. Centers for Disease Control. 1985. Recommendations for assisting in the prevention of perinatal transmission of human T-lymphotropic virus type III/lymphadenopathy-associated virus and acquired immunodeficiency syndrome. Morbid. Mortal. Wkly. Rep. 34:721-732.
28. American Academy of Pediatrics/American College of Obstetricians and Gynecologists. 1992. Guidelines for Perinatal Care, 3rd ed. American Academy of Pediatrics, Elk Grove, Ill.
29. Human Milk Banking Association of North America; Arnold, L.D.W., and M.R. Tully, eds. 1991. Guidelines for the Establishment and Operation of a Human Milk Bank. Human Milk Banking Association, West Hartford, Conn.
30. Brady, M.S., K.A. Rickard, J.F. Fitzgerald, and J.A. Lemons. 1986. Specialized formulas and feedings for infants with malabsorption or formula intolerance. J. Am. Diet. Assoc. 86:191-200.
31. Lemons, P., M. Stuart, and J.A. Lemons. 1986. Breast-feeding the premature infant. Clin. Perinatol. 13:111-122.
32. Lemons, P. 1983. Breast-feeding the premature newborn. Perinatal Press 7:83-88.
33. American Dietetic Association. 1991. Preparation of Formula for Infants: Guidelines for Health Care Facilities. American Dietetic Association, Chicago.
34. Grant, J., and S.C. Denne. 1991. Effect of intermittent versus continuous enteral feeding on energy expenditure in premature infants. J. Pediatr. 118:928-932.
35. Balistreri, W.F., and K. Bove. 1990. Hepatobiliary consequences of parenteral alimentation. Progr. Liver Dis. 9:567-601.
36. Dunn, L., S. Hulman, J. Weiner, and R. Kliegman. 1988. Beneficial effects of early hypochloric enteral feeding on neonatal gastrointestinal function: preliminary report of a randomized trial. J. Pediatr. 112:622-629.
37. Greene, H.L., K.M. Hambidge, R. Schanler, and R.C. Tsang. 1988. Guidelines for the use of vitamins, trace elements, calcium, magnesium, and phosphorus in infants and children receiving total parenteral nutrition: report of the Subcommittee on Pediatric Parenteral Nutrient Requirements from the Committee on Clinical Practice Issues of The American Society for Clinical Nutrition. Am. J. Clin. Nutr. 48:1324-1342.
38. Hanning, R.M., and S.H. Zlotkin. 1989. Amino acid and protein needs of the neonate: effects of excess and deficiency. Semin. Perinatol. 13:131-141.
39. Heird, W.C., W. Hay, R.A. Helms, M.C. Storm, S. Kashyap, and R.B. Dell. 1988. Pediatric parenteral amino acid mixture in low birth weight infants. Pediatrics 81:41-50.
40. Mayfield, S.R., J. Albrecht, L. Roberts, and C. Lair. 1989. The role of the nutritional support team in neonatal intensive care. Semin. Perinatol. 13:88-96.
41. Yowell-Warman, K., and P. Queen. 1989. Pediatric nutrition in the home. Pp. 142-174 in M. Hermann-Zaidins and R. Touger-Decker, eds. Nutrition Support in Home Health. Aspen Publishers, Inc., Rockville, Md.
42. Anderson, D.M. 1987. Nutrition care for the premature infant. Top. Clin. Nutr. 2:1-9.
43. Georgieff, M.K., and S.R. Sasanow. 1986. Nutritional assessment of the neonate. Clin. Perinatol. 13:73-89.
44. Ziegler, E.E. 1985. Nutritional management of the premature infant. Perinatol. Neonatol. 9:11-15.

45. Stave, V.S., S. Robbins, and A.B. Fletcher. 1979. A comparison of growth rates of premature infants prior to and after close nutritional monitoring. Clin. Proc. Children's Hosp. Natl. Med. Ctr. 35:171-180.
46. Lowe, W.W., T.A. Ciszek, and K.J. Gallaher. 1992. Comprehensive computerized neonatal intensive care unit data system including real-time, computer-generated daily progress notes. Pediatrics 89:62-66.
47. Dubowitz, L.M., V. Dubowitz, and C. Goldberg. 1970. Clinical assessment of gestational age in the newborn infant. J. Pediatr. 77:1-10.
48. Ballard, J.L., K.K. Novak, and M. Driver. 1979. A simplified score for assessment of fetal maturation of newly born infants. J. Pediatr. 95:769-774.
49. Sanders, M., M. Allen, G.R. Alexander, J. Yankowitz, J. Graeber, T.R.B. Johnson, and M.X. Repka. 1991. Gestational age assessment in preterm neonates weighing less than 1500 grams. Pediatrics 88:542-546.
50. Ballard, J.L., J.C. Khoury, K.Wedig, L. Wang, B.L. Eilers-Walsman, and R. Lipp. 1991. New Ballard Score, expanded to include extremely premature infants. J. Pediatr. 119:417-423.
51. Babson, S.G. 1970. Growth of low-birth-weight infants. J. Pediatr. 77:11-18.
52. Kaempf, J.W., C. Bonnabel, and W.W. Hay, Jr. 1989 2nd ed. Neonatal nutrition. Pp. 117-203 in G.B. Merenstein and S.L. Gardner, eds. Handbook of Neonatal Intensive Care. C.V. Mosby, St. Louis.
53. Dancis, J., J.R. O'Connell, and L.E. Holt, Jr. 1948. Grid for recording weight of premature infants. J. Pediatr. 33:570-572.
54. Babson, S.G., and G.I. Benda. 1976. Growth graphs for the clinical assessment of infants of varying gestational age. J. Pediatr. 89:814-820.
55. Gairdner, D., and Pearson, J. 1971. A growth chart for premature and other infants. Arch. Dis. Child. 46:783-787.
56. Lubchenco, L.O., C. Hansman, M. Dressler and E. Boyd. 1963. Intrauterine growth as estimated from live born birth-weight data at 24 to 42 weeks of gestation. Pediatrics 32:793-800.
57. Falkner, F. 1973. Long-term developmental studies: a critique. In Early Development. Research Publication of the Association for Research in Nervous and Mental Disease 51:416-418.
58. Ekblad, H., P. Kero, J. Takala, H. Korvenranta, and I. Valimaki. 1987. Water, sodium and acid-base balance in premature infants: therapeutical aspects. Acta Paediatr. Scand. 76:47-53.
59. Ross Planning Associates. 1988. Perspectives in Perinatal and Pediatric Design. Ross Laboratories, Columbus, Ohio.
60. American Dietetic Association; Kozlowski, B.W., and J.A. Powell. 1989. Position of The American Dietetic Association: nutrition services for children with special health care needs. J. Am. Diet. Assoc. 89:1133-1137.
61. Ehrenhaft, P.M., J.L. Wagner, and R.C. Herdman. 1989. Changing prognosis for very low birth weight infants. Obstet. Gynecol. 74:528-535.
62. Pittard, W.B. III, and D.M. Anderson. 1983. Neonatal nutrition training. J. Am. Diet. Assoc. 83:471-473.
63. Vanderveen, T., and R. Parks. 1981. ASHP supplemental standard and learning objectives for residency training in nutritional support pharmacy practice. Am. J. Hosp. Pharm. 38:1971-1973.
64. Brannon, M.E., and M.C. Egan. 1985. Nutrition in perinatal services: where are we? Perinatol. Neonatol. 9:11-20.

6

Providing for the Continuity of Nutritional Care

Delivering appropriate, coordinated nutrition services to cover the period beginning before conception and extending through infancy poses major challenges, especially because services typically are delivered at different sites and by different providers. For mothers or infants with special nutritional problems, continuity of care is especially important when a move is made from one site or level of care to another. Moreover, continuity of care may be especially difficult to achieve for the large numbers of women and families who do not have regular care providers, who experience shifts in their financial eligibility for services, who move between geographic areas (e.g., migrant workers), or who find it difficult to make the travel and child care arrangements necessary for acting on referrals or continuing with regular care.

Disadvantaged women have disproportionately high rates of preterm delivery, low-birth-weight infants, and other complications and adverse outcomes of pregnancy. Thus, efforts to overcome financial, cultural, language, and other barriers to effective communication and the continuity of nutritional care are especially valuable for such women and their families.

This chapter briefly reviews three approaches that have been proposed for improving communication and continuity of care:

- efforts to implement coordinated services, including *one-stop shopping* ("any local service system of integrated service delivery, where women and children can receive multiple health and/or social services at one site" (p. 6),[1]

- the integration of a well-designed, patient-carried health diary into the delivery of services, and
- the development and integration of computer-based patient records and systems.[2]

The second approach appears to be relatively easy to achieve; implementation of the other two would require greater commitment and effort, but it is reasonable to expect that such efforts would result in substantial improvements in care. Although these three approaches are intended to improve many aspects of overall health care, they may be especially useful in facilitating the improved delivery of nutrition services in support of maternal and infant health.

COORDINATED SERVICES

The coordination of health care services, food assistance, and social services can promote continuity of care and improve the integration of nutrition services into the care of pregnant and postpartum women. In 1986, the U.S. Departments of Health and Human Services (DHHS) and of Agriculture jointly sponsored a study of coordination between the Maternal and Child Health (MCH) Program of DHHS and the Special Supplemental Food Program for Women, Infants, and Children (WIC). The study concluded that coordinated care has the following objectives:

- a well developed referral system among the providers for each program
- the transfer of needed information between providers on an anticipatory basis
- avoidance of unnecessary duplication of functions between MCH and WIC programs, such as blood and anthropometric measurements
- the scheduling of services and different aspects of care such that they contribute to, rather than interfere with, the services and care being delivered in another program
- the design, content, and delivery of nutrition-related education components which do not contradict those delivered by another program serving the same patient
- improved case management, continuity of care and follow-up of shared clients (p. ii).[3]

The report of the first Ross Roundtable on Current Issues in Public Health, *The Role of MCH and WIC in the Delivery of Local Health Services*,[4] continued the dialogue on this topic: "The . . . greatest challenge is for all of us to realize that to meet needs, maternal and child health and nutrition must consist of more than WIC and more than Title V MCH nutrition services. We must be in collaboration—not in competition—with many other food, health, education, and welfare programs" (p. 84).[4]

The scope of coordinated care is described in two publications of the National Governors' Association;[5,6] the concept of *one-stop shopping* incorporates techniques for delivering such care. The three key elements of one-stop shopping[7] are (1) location of several health and human services at the same site, and development of procedures to integrate those services or to schedule several appointments sequentially so that the number of trips for care can be minimized; (2) establishment of a uniform application process for programs (e.g., only one form need be completed to determine eligibility for Medicaid, WIC, and a state-funded health care program); and (3) provision for handling applications for assistance at the site of care delivery (which may include assigning workers to distant sites—sometimes called "outposting" or "outstationing"[8]).

Many one-stop shoppping programs have been implemented. In Idaho, for example, a comprehensive prenatal health care model with one-stop shopping has led to expansion and improvement of WIC services; WIC, in turn, has helped attract and maintain participation in prenatal care.[9] Watkins and colleagues[10] describe a model program targeted to migrant women and their children that also emphasized coordinated services and follow-up.

With appropriate case coordination, there is considerable potential for promoting continuity of nutritional care in the public sector, especially since Medicaid funds can be used for perinatal nutrition services in many states.[11,12] In North Carolina, improved maternity care coordination for women on Medicaid has been associated with reductions in low birth weight, infant mortality, and medical care costs for newborns.[13]

PATIENT-CARRIED HEALTH DIARIES

The Omnibus Budget Reconciliation Act of 1989 required the Secretary of Health and Human Services to develop a model national maternal and child health handbook. Under the leadership of the Maternal and Child Health Bureau, a handbook called *Health Diary* is being developed (I. Heyman, Maternal and Child Health Bureau, personal communication, 1992). The *Health Diary* covers the period from conception through the second year after birth, providing basic information that includes recommendations on weight gain during pregnancy, healthful diets, and breastfeeding. It allows both the provider and the woman to record items of importance: any questions the woman may have, weights (of mother or baby, or both), advice given during the visit, date of the next appointment, and other matters. The diary is intended to enable the woman to be an active participant in her own and her infant's health care, encourage the adoption and maintenance of healthy behaviors, encourage the seeking of care, and enhance communication between providers and patients.

The functions described above for the health diary are similar to those suggested by Giglio and Papazian[14] for specially designed patient-carried records. (These records, which the woman keeps, are sometimes called "passports," "handbooks," or cards, depending on the form they take.) Studies suggest that several types of patient-carried records can help to promote continuity of care—for example, family-carried growth records,[15] antenatal cooperation cards,[16] adverse drug reaction cards,[17] and reminder cards for health maintenance procedures.[18] More elaborate patient-carried records have been reported to hold potential for improved care of migrants[10] and of homeless men.[19]

In 1990, 18 of the 54 states and territories reported the development of some type of patient-carried record,[1] and 8 of these had at least one kind of form for pregnant women (see, e.g., *Baby Your Baby Health Keepsake*[20]). There is at least one large-scale example of patient-carried records in operation: U.S. military health care facilities give their patients (including dependents of military personnel) their health records to carry. Although this system is not without problems,[21] its long history indicates that patient involvement can provide a useful means of improving continuity of care. The importance ascribed to patient-carried records by many in the public health field was highlighted in 1991: among the key actions in the Public Health Service's 1991 Plan to Strengthen Public Health in the United States[22] is the development of "maternal and child health handbooks to provide a home-based health record and basic information on health and development for pregnant women and new families" (p. 81).[22]

If health diaries with a strong nutritional component become widely used in maternal and infant care, improvements can be expected in both communication with patients and the continuity of nutritional care. For maximum effectiveness, clinicians need to use the health diary to identify and record nutrition-related information during health care visits, encourage the woman to use it at home, and ask her to bring it to office visits. In this way, reasonable tracking of the woman's nutritional care and progress can occur even if the woman must see many different providers at different sites.

COMPUTER-BASED PATIENT RECORDS AND SYSTEMS

The Institute of Medicine Committee on Improving the Patient Record has recommended the following: "Health care professionals and organizations should adopt the computer-based patient record as the standard for medical and all other records related to patient care" (p. 6).[2] That committee views the future patient record as offering broader functions than those provided by current record systems:

> The future patient record will be a computer-based, multimedia record . . . that offers access (availability, convenience, speed, reliability, and ease of use), quality, security, flexibility, connectivity, and efficiency. In addition, future patient records will provide new functions through links to other databases and decision support tools (p. 135).[2]

The committee's final report, *The Computer-Based Patient Record: An Essential Technology for Health Care*,[2] contains a strategic implementation plan, advocates prompt development and implementation of the system (within the decade), and addresses measures to protect the patient's confidentiality.

Such a system would have special utility for the maternal and child health population[2] and would allow great strides to be made in nutritional care. Individualized nutritional care plans could be developed and updated readily for women and their infants—including those who require complex care because of health problems or disabilities. Only authorized care providers would have access to the information entered into the data base concerning the results of nutritional assessments, the setting of specific nutritional objectives, changes in the patient's status, and so forth. Transfer of information about the mother relevant to the care of the infant could be handled easily, and advanced features could facilitate decision making in complex situations, such as the nutritional care of very-low-birth-weight infants.

SUMMARY

Improved delivery of nutritional care in support of maternal and infant health requires concrete measures to improve communication and continuity of care. Promising approaches with widespread applicability include expansion of the one-stop shopping concept, development and widespread use of patient-carried health diaries that have a strong nutritional component, and development and implementation of computer-based patient record systems. Until such approaches become widely available, providers can use forms, referrals, supportive personnel (e.g., case managers and nurse home visitors), and other linkages to foster improved continuity of care.

REFERENCES

1. Association of Maternal and Child Health Programs. 1990. Building on the Basics: Four Approaches to Enhancing MCH Service Delivery. Association of Maternal and Child Health Programs, Washington, D.C.
2. Institute of Medicine; Dick, R.S., and E.B. Steen, eds. 1991. The Computer-Based Patient Record: An Essential Technology for Health Care. National Academy Press, Washington, D.C.
3. Pindus, N., B. Duggar, and C. Schulz. 1986. Improving MCH/WIC Coordination: Final Report and Guide to Good Practices. Professional Management Associates, Inc., Rockville, Md.
4. Dwyer, J.T., ed. 1987. The Role of MCH and WIC in the Delivery of Local Health Services. Report of the First Ross Roundtable on Current Issues in Public Health. Ross Laboratories, Columbus, Ohio.
5. Hill, I.T., and Bennett, T. 1990. Enhancing the Scope of Prenatal Services: Strategies for Improving State Perinatal Programs. National Governors' Association, Washington, D.C.
6. Hill, I.T., and J. Breyel. 1989. Coordinating Prenatal Care. National Governors' Association, Washington, D.C.
7. Macro Systems, Inc. 1990. One-Stop Shopping for Perinatal Services: Identification and Assessment of Implementation Methodologies. National Center for Education in Maternal and Child Health, Washington, D.C.
8. Hill, I.T. 1988. Reaching Women Who Need Prenatal Care. National Governors' Association, Washington, D.C.
9. Machala, M., and M.W. Miner. 1991. Piecing together the crazy quilt of prenatal care. Public Health Rep. 106:353-360.
10. Watkins, E.L., K. Larson, C. Harlan, and S. Young. 1990. A model program for providing health services for migrant farmworker mothers and children. Public Health Rep. 105:567-575.
11. Caldwell, M. 1991. Financing nutrition programs. Pp. 289-302 in C. Sharbaugh, ed. Call to Action: Better Nutrition for Mothers, Children, and Families. National Center for Education in Maternal and Child Health, Washington, D.C.
12. Summer, L. 1991. Working Together: A Guide to Coordinating WIC and Medicaid Services. Center on Budget and Policy Priorities, Washington, D.C.

13. Buescher, P.A., M.S. Roth, D. Williams, and C.M. Goforth. 1991. An evaluation of the impact of maternity care coordination on Medicaid birth outcomes in North Carolina. Am. J. Public Health 81:1625-1629.
14. Giglio, R.J., and B. Papazian. 1986. Acceptance and use of patient-carried health records. Med. Care 24:1084-1092.
15. Young, S.A., M. Kaufman, K. Larson, and E.L. Watkins. 1990. Family-carried growth records: a tool for providing continuity of care for migrant children. Public Health Nurs. 7:209-214.
16. Draper, J., S. Field, H. Thomas, and M.J. Hare. 1986. Should women carry their antenatal records? Br. Med. J. 292:603.
17. Hannaford, P.D. 1986. Adverse drug reaction cards carried by patients. Br. Med. J. 292:1109-1112.
18. Turner, R.C., L.E. Waivers, and K. O'Brien. 1990. The effect of patient-carried reminder cards on the performance of health maintenance measures. Arch. Intern. Med. 150:645-647.
19. Reuler, J.B., and J.R. Balazs. 1991. Portable medical record for the homeless mentally ill. Br. Med. J. 303:446.
20. Utah Department of Health, Family Health Services Division. 1990. Baby Your Baby Health Keepsake. Utah Department of Health, Salt Lake City.
21. Curtis, M.R. 1989. The patient-carried medical record. J. Qual. Assurance 11(1):34.
22. Assistant Secretary for Health's Public Health Service Task Force to Strengthen Public Health in the United States. 1991. A plan to strengthen public health in the United States. Public Health Rep. 106 (Suppl. 1):1-86.

7

Closing Remarks and Recommendations

Nutrition clearly makes a difference to the health of women, to outcomes of pregnancy and lactation, and to the health, growth, and development of infants. Of the many contenders for health care resources, nutrition services warrant substantial attention and support. This chapter summarizes underlying themes of the report and presents the committee's major recommendations.

It is customary to consider nutrition services in relation to a specific type of patient (e.g., a pregnant or a breastfeeding woman) as has been done in this report. However, the committee preferred to consider the delivery of nutrition services in relation to growing families rather than specific types of patients. It agreed that such delivery could be improved by five general measures:

- explicit recognition by all health team members of the essential role of nutrition in promoting health and growth;
- a team effort to provide nutritional care that is individualized and patient centered;
- the active involvement of families or other supportive persons in the formulation and implementation of a nutritional care plan;
- the implementation of concrete steps to achieve continuity of nutritional care; and
- nutrition education and training for health care providers.

Each of these measures requires adequate allocation of time and financial resources to allow clinicians to interact with, teach, and learn from other health care providers, the patient, and family members. The following sections provide further clarification of most of the measures mentioned above.

MEASURES FOR IMPROVING NUTRITIONAL CARE

Patient-Centered, Individualized Care

Patient-centered nutritional care requires an individualized approach. This means that a nutritional assessment should precede decisions concerning nutritional care. The term *nutritional assessment* covers a wide range of activities, not all of which are appropriate for all individuals. However, basic nutritional assessment for all patients encompasses the measurement of height or length and weight, the determination of hemoglobin or hematocrit values, and the assessment of dietary practices. Abnormal findings may indicate the need for more thorough assessment and intensive nutritional care.

Appropriate patient-centered care often requires that the health care team seek assistance for the patient from outside sources, generally through referral. This assistance may involve, for example, transport of neonates with complex nutrition and feeding requirements to a neonatal intensive care unit; referral to a center for the treatment of inborn errors of metabolism or diabetes mellitus; referral to the Special Supplemental Food Program for Women, Infants, and Children (WIC) for food supplementation and nutrition education; or referral to a program for the treatment of eating disorders. Structured procedures are needed to facilitate implementation of the referral, to track whether appropriate follow-up has occurred, and to indicate how care is to be altered, if at all, as a result.

If transportation or other logistical difficulties make it impossible to arrange for a referral or to incorporate the required specialist into the health care team, the health care provider is urged to consult with a dietitian who specializes in either maternal or neonatal nutrition and with other specialists as needed.

Family Involvement in Care

Support from family or friends may have a strong impact on how well the woman or her infant, or both, are nourished. Improving maternal weight gain, addressing breastfeeding problems, or initiating an alternative feeding method (such as tube feeding) often calls for the involvement of supportive persons in developing and implementing the care plan. For breastfeeding women, influential friends may need to be involved, as well as the woman's partner. To lay the foundation for appropriate home care of premature or sick infants, those who will be the principal caregivers at home should be involved in nurturing and feeding the infant in the hospital. They also need guidance to form realistic expectations for the infant's development and to understand how development relates to the progression of feedings.

Team Care

For healthy women or infants, the minimal team comprises the patient and her health care provider (physician or midwife). The efforts of nurses, dietitians, social workers, and health educators increase the potential to address common problems that interfere with normal nutrition; they can also increase the patient's understanding of healthful diets and how to achieve them. If a dietitian is not a member of the practice or of the health team, the committee recommends that an active, formalized relationship be established with a dietitian for periodic in-service education, consultation about patient care, and information about useful nutrition-related resources.

A coordinated, multidisciplinary health care team is essential to deal with complex nutrition problems. Depending on the nature of the problem, such a team would ordinarily include the physician, nurses, a dietitian, and an assortment of other providers such as a pharmacist, social worker, breastfeeding specialist, and physical therapist. For families that have difficulty dealing with the medical system because of language or cultural barriers, learning disorders, or other reasons, a trained peer counselor may help serve as a bridge between them and the rest of the health care team (see *Nutrition During Pregnancy and Lactation: An Implementation Guide*[1]).

Nutritional Care Plans

Using the nutritional assessment as a base, a nutritional care plan should be developed for all pregnant and lactating women and for infants. For many, the care plan will simply call for routine monitoring and one or two specific objectives for improving or maintaining nutritional status. However, many situations and health problems call for more detailed care plans. An essential method for communicating the care plan is thorough documentation in the permanent medical record. The specification of follow-up care is a standard component of care plans but one that needs to be emphasized.

Education and Training of Practitioners

For basic nutritional care before, during, and after pregnancy, the publication *Nutrition During Pregnancy and Lactation: An Implementation Guide*,[1] provides sound guidance and sources of supplementary information for practicing physicians, midwives, nurses, dietitians, and other care providers. The use of that guidebook can be enhanced by short training sessions.

For the more complex nutritional care of pregnant and lactating women with health problems and of infants with special needs, providers should have specialized training or closely supervised experience. Specialized training requires both didactic and clinical multidisciplinary learning experiences over weeks or months. Moreover, because of rapid developments in maternal and neonatal nutrition, members of the health care team need access to periodic updates through conferences or short courses.

RECOMMENDATIONS

This report contains eight key recommendations:

- **Basic, patient-centered, individualized nutritional care should be integrated into the primary care of every woman and infant–beginning prior to conception and extending throughout the period of breastfeeding.** The components of such care are defined in this document and described in greater detail in *Nutrition During Pregnancy and Lactation: An Implementation Guide.*

• **All primary care providers should have the knowledge and skills necessary to screen for nutritional problems, assess nutritional status, provide basic nutritional guidance, and implement basic nutritional care.** This knowledge and the development of these skills should be part of the education of primary care providers. Several reports have indicated that nutrition education in medical schools and clinical residencies is often inadequate.[2-6] Medical schools, accreditation bodies, and professional organizations should address these deficiencies. The committee recommends that practitioners who need to develop these skills participate in training sessions based on the content of *Nutrition During Pregnancy and Lactation: An Implementation Guide.*

• **Nutritional care should be documented in the permanent medical record.** Documentation may be simplified through the use of forms or computerized systems.

• **When health problems that benefit from special nutritional care are identified, there should be consultation with and often referral to an experienced registered dietitian or other appropriate specialists.** Ongoing communication and cooperation between the primary care provider and special care provider(s) are essential to maintain quality care.

• **Attention should be directed toward aspects of care that have been seriously neglected: nutritional care prior to conception, care in support of breastfeeding, and ensuring the continuity of nutritional care despite changes in providers.** To achieve the latter, the committee urges continuing efforts to coordinate Maternal and Child Health programs with WIC programs, to implement the one-stop shopping concept, and to adopt the use of patient-carried health diaries with a strong nutritional component. Moreover, it urges experts in maternal and infant nutrition to become involved in the development of the computer-based patient record as described in a recent Institute of Medicine report.[7]

• **Action should be taken to make appropriate policy and structural changes for the promotion and support of breastfeeding.** Employers, for example, could be encouraged to eliminate barriers to breastfeeding in the workplace. This might involve allowing sufficient time for the mother to feed her infant or pump her breasts and the provision of a private area for such activities; it might also involve provision of a pump and refrigeration or the establishment of a nearby infant care center.

• At many sites, a major barrier to the implementation of the recommendations in this document is the lack of financial coverage for the time or personnel involved in providing nutrition services. **Where not already in place, mechanisms should be established to pay for basic and special nutrition services in both the public and private sectors.** For instance, time for the provision of basic nutrition services should be factored into cost-based reimbursement calculations for primary care. Special nutritional care should be a reimbursable item.

• **Cost-effective strategies for implementing the nutritional care recommended in this report should be developed and tested.** For example, studies are needed to identify effective methods of incorporating nutrition services in home visits and to clarify the costs and benefits of such visits at various points during and after pregnancy.

REFERENCES

1. Institute of Medicine. 1992. Nutrition During Pregnancy and Lactation: An Implementation Guide. Report of the Subcommittee for a Clinical Applications Guide, Committee on Nutritional Status During Pregnancy and Lactation, Food and Nutrition Board. National Academy Press, Washington, D.C.
2. Boker, J.R., R.L. Weinsier, C.M. Brooks, and A.K. Olson. 1990. Components of effective clinical-nutrition training: a national survey of graduate medical education (residency) programs. Am. J. Clin. Nutr. 52:568-571.
3. Feldman, E.B. 1991. Educating physicians in nutrition–a view of the past, the present, and the future. Am. J. Clin. Nutr. 54:618-622.
4. National Research Council. 1985. Nutrition Education in U.S. Medical Schools. Committee on Nutrition in Medical Education, Food and Nutrition Board. National Academy Press, Washington, D.C.
5. Weinsier, R.L., J.R. Boker, E.B. Feldman, M.S. Read, and C.M. Brooks. 1986. Nutrition knowledge of senior medical students: a collaborative study of southeastern medical schools. Am. J. Clin. Nutr. 43:959-965.
6. Weinsier, R.L., J.R. Boker, C.M. Brooks, R.F. Kushner, A.K. Olson, D.A. Mark, S.T. St. Jeor, V.A. Stallings, M. Winick, D. Heber, and W.J. Visek. 1991. Nutrition training in graduate medical (residency) education: a survey of selected training programs. Am. J. Clin. Nutr. 54:957-962.
7. Institute of Medicine; Dick, R.S., and E.B. Steen, eds. 1991. The Computer-Based Patient Record: An Essential Technology for Health Care. National Academy Press, Washington, D.C.

Index